Pathways in paediatr

Pathways in paediatrics

B. G. Loftus
Department of Paediatrics, University College
Hospital, Galway, Ireland

Edward Arnold
A member of the Hodder Headline Group
LONDON BOSTON MELBOURNE AUCKLAND

First published in Great Britain 1995 by Edward Arnold, a division of Hodder Headline PLC, 338 Euston Road, London NW1 3BH

Distributed by Little, Brown and Company, 34 Beacon Street, Boston, MA 02108

British Library Cataloguing in Publication Data

Loftus, Brendan Gerald
Pathways in Paediatrics
I. Title
618.92

ISBN 0-340-59036-x

Typeset in 10/11 pt Times by Anneset, Weston-super-Mare, Avon. Printed and bound in Great Britain by Mackays of Chatham PLC, Kent.

Contents

Contributors vii
Preface ix
Acknowledgements xi

1 The clinical process in paediatrics 1

Part I Acute presentations
2 Acute diarrhoea 9
3 Acute vomiting 18
4 Bleeding and bruising 25
5 The collapsed child 32
6 Child abuse 37
7 Cough 46
8 Crying 52
9 Dyspnoea 58
10 Fever 65
11 Haematuria 72
12 Jaundice 77
13 Limp 87
14 Oedema 91
15 Poisoning 96
16 Seizure 103
17 Sudden infant death/apparent life-threatening event 112
18 Stridor 119

Part II Outpatient presentations
19 Abnormal puberty 127
20 Asthma outpatient management 135
21 Behavioural problems 142
22 Chronic diarrhoea 149
23 Constipation 155

24 Cystic fibrosis outpatient management 163
25 Developmental delay 169
26 Diabetes mellitus outpatient management 176
27 Nocturnal enuresis 180
28 Failure to thrive 186
29 Fits and funny turns 192
30 Headache 199
31 Murmur 205
32 Neonatal cholestasis 217
33 Pallor 229
34 Recurrent abdominal pain 233
35 Recurrent infections 238
36 Short stature 245
37 Skin rash 255

Index 263

Contributors

Dr Kevin Connolly MB, FRCPI, DCH, Consultant Paediatrician, Portiuncula Hospital, Ballinasloe, Co. Galway.
(Chaps 8, 17, 21)

Professor Brendan Drumm MB, FRCPI, DCH, Paediatric Gastroenterologist, Our Lady's Hospital for Sick Children, Dublin 12.
(Chaps 2, 12, 32)

Dr Desmond Duff MB, FRCPI, DCH, Paediatric Cardiologist, Our Lady's Hospital for Sick Children, Dublin 12.
(Chap. 31)

Dr Kevin Dunne MB, MRCP, DCH, Consultant Paediatrician, University College Hospital, Galway.
(Chaps 25, 30)

Professor Denis Gill MB, BSc, FRCPI, DCH, Paediatric Nephrologist, The Children's Hospital, Temple Street, Dublin 1.
(Chaps 5, 11, 27)

Dr John Gleeson MB, MRCPI, DCH, Consultant Paediatrician, Sligo General Hospital, Ireland.
(Chaps 7, 9, 35)

Dr Norma Goggin MB, DCH, Paediatric Registrar, Our Lady's Hospital for Sick Children, Dublin 12.
(Chap. 2)

Dr Siobhan Gormally MD, MRCP, DCH, Lecturer in Paediatrics, Our Lady's Hospital for Sick Children, Dublin 12.
(Chaps 2, 12, 32)

Dr Owen Hensey MB, BSc, FRCPI, Consultant Paediatrician, The Children's Hospital, Temple Street, Dublin.
(Chap. 6)

Professor Hilary Hoey MD, FRCPI, DCH, Paediatric Endocrinologist, National Children's Hospital, Hardcourt Street, Dublin 2.
(Chaps 19, 36)

Professor Peter Kearney MB, BSc, FRCP, FRCPI, DCH, Consultant Paediatrician, Cork Regional Hospital, Ireland.
(Chaps 4, 23, 34)

Dr Peter Keenan MB, FRCPI, DCH, Consultant in Accident & Emergency, The Children's Hospital, Temple Street, Dublin.
(Chaps 13, 15, 18)

Professor B Gerard Loftus MD, FRCPI, DCH, Consultant Paediatrician, University College Hospital, Galway, Ireland.
(Chaps 1, 3, 5, 10, 14, 16, 20, 22, 24, 26, 28, 29, 33, 37)

Preface

Common sense ain't all that common

Mark Twain.

Most diagnostic and treatment decisions in paediatrics are based on simple clinical evaluation. The major textbooks are system or disease based, leaving a need for a symptom based text to assist the development of clinical problem solving skills. *Pathways in Paediatrics* is an attempt to fill this gap.

The common, important presentations in emergency and outpatient practice were selected and strategies developed for assessment and management. In some instances the clinical problem is primarily diagnostic, in others therapeutic – the sections are structured accordingly. This text cannot be comprehensive or definitive, but aims to help senior undergraduates and paediatric residents develop an orderly approach to clinical problems.

As with any multiple contributor text there are some inconsistencies in style, approach and depth. I hope that this will serve to maintain interest rather than induce confusion. Inevitably there may be omissions and inaccuracies and for these, I apologise. Readers' suggestions and criticisms are welcomed.

BG Loftus
1994

Acknowledgements

Professor John Price helped develop the framework for the book. I am indebted to the contributors for their support with this project. Debbie Monroe typed and processed all the text – several times!

For Denise

1 The clinical process in paediatrics

Introduction

In paediatrics, as in other areas of medicine, the patient presentation is an ill structured problem. Following brief analysis and incorporating the clinician's perceptions and key observations, an initial concept is formed. This initial concept basically tells us what kind of problem we are facing and this is further refined to enable a diagnostic hypothesis to be generated. We then formulate an enquiry strategy to confirm or reject the hypothesis. The enquiry strategy can be divided into the 'search', where open-ended questions, focusing directly on the presenting complaint, are formulated to confirm or reject the generated hypothesis, and the 'scan' where routine details of past history, family history and systems review are obtained. The available data are then summarised and subjected to deductive logic. The clinical examination follows. The experienced clinician will always look for specific items related to the presentation.

Most experienced clinicians generate a diagnostic hypothesis within minutes of initial patient contact and this should be refined to a working diagnosis after the clinical examination. Laboratory investigations in paediatrics are often unproductive in terms of making a specific diagnosis. Treatment decisions are based on the consultation, working diagnosis and laboratory investigations. Treatment can be viewed as patient education to encourage compliance with a prescribed regime and with behaviour modification. Approximately 40 per cent of the consultation will be devoted to patient education. If patient education is inadequately supplied, the consultation will have been wasted.

Presentation

Children will rarely attend a physician on their own. The parent who brings the child will have formed the opinion that the child is ill and in need of medical attention. One of the particular problems in paediatrics is that much of the history is second hand and in infants and young children, there will be no collateral history from the patient. The symptoms may present in a particularly ill structured fashion. Parental experience, expectation and current upsets in family dynamics may well have influenced the presentation. Always bear in mind that the patient is the one with the problem. An open-ended question such as 'What is worrying you most about your child?' will help bring forward the key presenting symptoms. Listen carefully and try to avoid bias and errors in translation. As you listen, observe the child and the parent. Try at all times to be objective.

Initial concept

The initial concept will be based on the key observations and facts presented to the clinician. It should be flexible and allowed to develop as the consultation proceeds. Further questioning will allow the initial concept to be encapsulated and to provide a narrower focus for diagnostic hypothesis generation. For example, 'a 6-week-old child with vomiting' presents a bewilderingly long list of possible diagnoses whereas 'a 6-week-old with projectile vomiting' or 'a 6-week-old with fever, anorexia and vomiting' will push the diagnostic decision making in a very different direction.

Hypothesis generation

This is essentially a series of educated guesses as to a diagnosis which fits best with the initial concept. For instance, the previously described 6-week-old child with vomiting will cause an initial series of hypotheses to be generated and as further information becomes available the diagnostic possibilities can be narrowed down. Pyloric stenosis is very probable if the child has projectile vomiting and is hungry immediately afterwards, whereas gastroenteritis would be the more likely diagnosis if there was concomitant diarrhoea and a history of recent contact within the family. The initial hypothesis must always be tentative and it is very important not to be too fixed on a diagnosis too early in the process, as one can then unconsciously lead the patient and censor the data to sustain an incorrect diagnosis. Always leave a diagnostic loophole large enough to crawl back through.

Enquiry strategy

This part of the consultation has essentially two components. The first is the search for a specific diagnosis. Use open ended questions initially, directly focusing on the presenting complaint. Define the reason for the consultation, the onset of the symptom, the events at the onset of the symptom and the quality and intensity of the symptom. Associated symptoms should be elicited and also the temporal progression of the symptom and the sequence of the various presenting symptoms. Where possible, define the localisation of the symptom, the preceding events and factors which relieve or aggravate the symptom. Keep asking questions until you can imagine having the symptom yourself. This is the most productive part of the history.

The second part is the 'scan'. The past history is reviewed. Routine questions would include the birth history, immunisation status, developmental progress and previous hospitalisation. Specific queries would be raised depending on the diagnostic hypothesis. For example, in a child with possible cystic fibrosis, enquiry as to previous respiratory infections would be very important. The family history, social history and system review are covered briefly in this mode. As medical students, we are encouraged to take comprehensive family and social history. This rarely produces new information that is important to the diagnostic process but the information gleaned may be important in making decisions regarding treatment and in influencing the method of patient education.

Having completed the enquiry strategy, further questioning may be appropriate, depending on the influence of the information gained on the working hypothesis. It is helpful at this time to summarise for the patient and the parent your concept of the history to date, e.g. 'So you are telling me that James was well until two days ago, when he lost all interest in eating, began to vomit everything that he drank and developed a fever'.

Clinical skills

The experienced clinician will apply deductive logic, intuition and overview to the available information. These skills come naturally with experience and are difficult to categorise, in much the same way that the skills required for riding a bicycle are difficult to describe in print. The clinician will draw on previous experience for pattern recognition and, particularly in difficult cases, a reservoir of basic science knowledge to formulate a working diagnosis and to give him a good idea of what physical findings he will be seeking. The clinical examination may be considered a ritual which is modified depending on the history and which incorporates a scan for unexpected findings. Every clinician will develop his own routine for examination and once you have developed a satisfactory, comprehensive routine – stick to it!

Clinical examination occasionally produces surprises but in general contributes surprisingly little to the diagnostic process. In infants and toddlers, examination may be resisted and the quality of the information available is limited. The most valuable information from the clinical examination is usually obtained from inspection of the child as he sits on the parent's knee or plays around the room. Remember the advice, 'If you don't look you won't see, if you don't listen you won't hear, if you don't sniff you won't smell'.

Investigation

'Tests' are often of little value in the diagnostic process. Investigations do become more important with rarer diseases and particularly at tertiary level consultation. Investigations can be viewed as producing four types of information:

- evidence for or against the diagnosis.
- assessment of the severity of the illness.
- reassurance by excluding more serious diagnosis.
- a specific influence on management.

Always ask yourself, is this going to produce useful information? When planning individual investigations consider the following.

- sensitivity – how confident am I that this test will detect the condition I suspect?
- specificity – if this test is positive, is the disease definitely present?
- The relevance to patient care – is the result of this test going to alter the patient's management or give information with regard to prognosis?
- The benefit-to-risk ratio – is this test going to be very expensive; does it take a long time to get a result; will this simply delay appropriate treatment of the patient's condition; will this test be uncomfortable?

Use tests like a rifle, not a shotgun – one shot at a time, with precision. Curiosity is not an indication for investigation – curiosity kills not only cats but also diagnostic accuracy.

The treatment decision

When we have reached a firm diagnosis we need to communicate this and its implications to the patient and parent. Frequently, where serious disease is excluded, management is largely expectant and reassurance is the treatment applied. This scenario is common and occasionally irritating, particularly out of hours. It is worth remembering that whilst we treat many conditions, anxiety is one of the few that we can cure. If the consultation was deemed inappropriate or alarmist, always remember that 'difficult people have difficulties' – there may be another agenda.

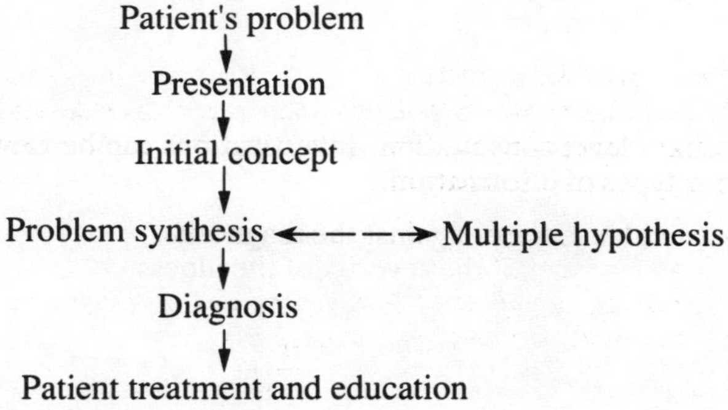

Fig. 1.1 Pathway for the clinical process

The treatment decision will involve rational prescribing. Patient education is vital so that the condition is understood and the rationale of any prescribed medication or behaviour modification is clear. This will give the greatest chance of ensuring patient compliance. Over a third of the consultation time will be spent on patient education and it is remarkable how ineffective this is sometimes. In an outpatient setting, parents will remember perhaps 30–40 per cent of the key information that is conveyed. Allow time for parents to ask questions and ask them to summarise what you have just told them – you will be surprised! Written information is very helpful and some clinicians provide tape recordings of the consultation for the parents to review at leisure. This part of the consultation is time well spent. In the words of an eminent paediatric surgeon, 'The child with abdominal pain can be dealt with during a single forty-minute consultation, two twenty-minute consultations, or four ten-minute consultations'.

Useful literature

- *Developing clinical problem-solving skills,* H. Barrows and G. Pickell (Norton Medical Books, 1991)
- *Paediatric clinical examination,* 2nd edition, D. Gill and N. O'Brien (Churchill Livingstone, 1993)

PART I

Acute Presentations

2 Acute diarrhoea

Acute 'diarrhoea' is one of the most frequent problems encountered by paediatricians. The normal bowel frequency for breastfed babies can vary from three times per week to twelve times per day. In the toddler age group, several bowel motions per day containing food particles may be normal in a child who is otherwise thriving. 'Diarrhoea' therefore is defined as an increase in the frequency, fluidity and volume of faeces as a result of deranged intestinal electrolyte and water transport.

Acute diarrhoea is a common cause of morbidity in childhood and remains a major reason for admission to paediatric units worldwide. There has been a dramatic fall in mortality in developed countries from acute diarrhoea in recent years. This is attributed to improvements in public health and personal hygiene and more recently to a reduction in the incidence of hypernatraemic dehydration. Acute diarrhoea remains a major contributor to both morbidity and mortality in the developing countries. During the first three years of life, a child in Africa or Asia experiences an estimated four acute, severe episodes of diarrhoea. One to 4 per cent of these episodes are fatal and each year approximately 5 million infants and children die in Latin America, Asia and Africa of diarrhoeal dehydration.

Acute diarrhoea may result from a variety of infectious agents, medications, toxins and dietary indiscretions (Table 2.1). However, the majority of cases are secondary to infection from viruses, bacteria or parasites. Rotavirus is the single most important pathogen because of its frequency and because it is associated with severe dehydration. Most outbreaks of acute diarrhoea in developed countries are viral in origin. Viruses account for 30 per cent of cases of infectious diarrhoea in developing countries. In contrast as many as 45 per cent of episodes in developing countries are caused by bacterial infection. The mechanisms of spread of bacterial and viral enteric infections are the same throughout the world. Most are spread by person-to-person contact (the faecal-oral route). Contaminated water and food may also be important in developing countries.

Assessment (Fig. 2.1)

History

The term 'diarrhoea' means different things to different people and therefore the number, volume and characteristics of the stools being passed must be documented. Very high volumes of watery fluid,

Table 2.1 Causes of acute diarrhoea

1. Acute gastroenteritis	
Viral	**Parasitic**
Rotavirus	*Giardia lamblia*
Norwalk virus	Cryptosporidium
Enteric-type adenovirus	*Entamoeba histolytica*
Astrovirus	*Dientamoeba fragilis*
Calcivirus	*Blastocytosis hominis*
Bacterial	
Campylobacter jejuni	
Salmonella enteritidis	
Shigella sonnei/flexneri	
Enterotoxic *E. coli*	
Enterohaemorrhagic *E. coli*	
Enteropathogenic *E. coli*	
Yersinia enterocolitica	
Clostridium difficile	
Aeromonas hydrophilia	
Plesimonas shigelloides	
Vibrio species	
2. Toxin mediated food poisoning	
Staphylococcus aureus	
Clostridium perfringens	
Bacillus cereus	
3. Systemic infection	
4. Antibiotic associated	

not affected by fasting, point towards a secretory diarrhoea as seen in enterotoxin producing *E. coli* or cholera. Rotavirus and cryptosporidium produce offensive, malodorous stools.

Valuable information concerning the magnitude of fluid loss that has occurred can be obtained in the history. It is difficult to quantify volume of stool and vomitus but the frequency of urinary outputs may provide some appreciation of the severity of dehydration. It is easier to quantify intake as many children will already have been commenced on clear fluid by their parents at the time of presentation.

The presence of systemic symptoms may provide clues to the aetiology of an acute diarrhoeal episode. More than 60 per cent of children presenting with rotavirus will have a history of recent or concurrent respiratory illness. A history of abrupt onset of symptoms with blood and mucus in the stools in association with abdominal pain, tenesmus and fever is suggestive of a bacterial infection. Arthralgia and arthritis may sometimes accompany salmonella infection.

Several risk factors are of importance in the aetiology of acute infectious diarrhoea. A comprehensive history should therefore include information regarding socioeconomic factors and education level of the family. Both are known to influence hygienic practices and sanitation conditions, which in turn play a role in transmission of infection. Children may have had previous hospital admissions for similar problems. A history of exposure to other individuals with diarrhoea is also pertinent. Recent travel to foreign countries is relevant in cases of infection with shigella or enterotoxigenic *E. coli*, and amoebiasis, cholera and giardiasis.

Clinical evaluation

The initial clinical assessment of a child with acute diarrhoea includes the documentation of heart rate, blood pressure and temperature. This information, together with an assessment of their state of hydration, will dictate the need for immediate resuscitative measures. The most accurate assessment of dehydration is made by comparing pre-illness weight with present weight. Other useful indicators include the child's general appearance and alertness, urinary output, tissue turgor, temperature of hands and feet, capillary refill time, appearance of the eyes and mucous membranes and fontanelle tension.

Dehydration is graded as mild, moderate or severe based on these signs. In mild dehydration, 3–5 per cent of body weight has been lost in fluid. Mild dehydration may result only in thirst with no abnormal physical findings. In contrast, 10 per cent or greater weight loss occurs in severe dehydration. This may be associated with signs of circulatory failure reflected in a decreased or absent urinary output, a rapid, sometimes impalpable pulse and a low blood pressure. The child may appear cold, mottled, sweaty or cyanosed. Abdominal examination is often unhelpful in these children. Estimates of degree of dehydration based solely on clinical findings tend to exaggerate the deficit.

Investigations

The majority of children with acute diarrhoea will have spontaneous resolution of symptoms within 24–48 hours. Those with minimal or mild dehydration can be treated at home and do not require further investigation. Children with moderate or severe dehydration require hospital admission to correct the fluid deficit that exists and to investigate the underlying cause of diarrhoea.

The total peripheral blood white cell count may be normal, decreased or increased. A relative lymphocytosis is seen with viral

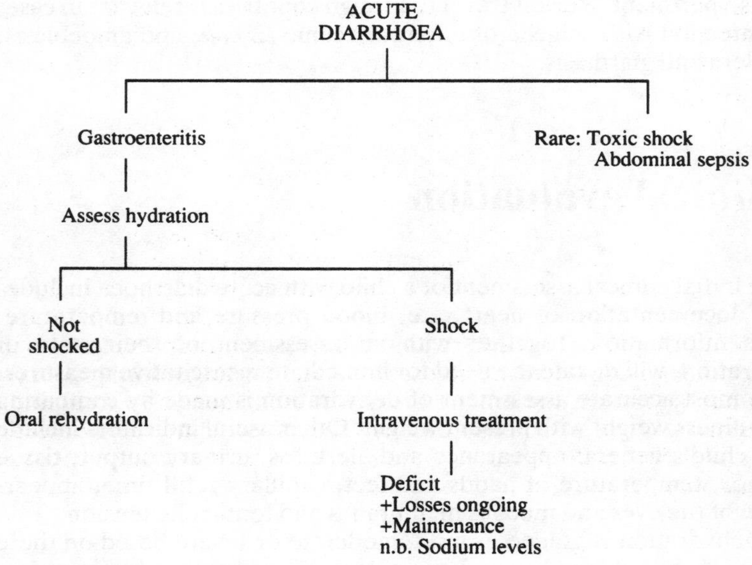

Fig. 2.1 Pathway for diagnosis and management of acute diarrhoea

infections. Increased 'band' forms on a blood film suggest shigella, salmonella, or campylobacter infection rather than *E. coli* or viral diarrhoea. Blood cultures may yield positive results in cases of invasive bacterial infection.

The measurement of urea and electrolytes, creatinine, serum osmolarity and blood pH status is important in any child who is moderately or severely dehydrated. The serum sodium can be normal, decreased or increased depending on the relative losses of water and electrolytes. Isotonic dehydration (serum sodium 130–150 mmol/l) is the common finding in children with acute diarrhoea and is characterised by a proportional loss of sodium and water. The extracellular fluid remains isotonic. There is therefore no osmotic gradient between the intra- and extracellular compartments.

Hyponatraemic dehydration (serum sodium < 130 mmol/l) results when there is a disproportionate loss of sodium over water or when water intake exceeds that of sodium. The hypotonicity of the extracellular fluid results in an osmotically induced movement of fluid from the extracellular compartment into the cells leading to even further depletion of fluid from the extracellular compartment. In hypernatraemic dehydration (serum sodium > 150 mmol/l) relatively less solute than body water is lost. The increase in osmolarity of the extracellular fluid results in a movement of fluid out of the cells leading to a depletion of intracellular fluid volume.

Urinary output, specific gravity and osmolarity are also important indices in dehydration. Concentrated urine occurs as a response to dehydration. This may progress to oliguria in children with severe dehydration.

Stool analysis can provide useful clinical information regarding the aetiology of acute diarrhoea. The presence of polymorphonuclear leucocytes in a stool are suggestive of bacterial infection. Rectal swabs or stool specimens can be cultured either to identify common bacterial pathogens such as *Campylobacter jejuni*, salmonella or shigella. Stool cultures should be repeated on several occasions. Specific culture media may be required, e.g. for campylobacter and yersinia but many viruses do not grow readily in cell culture. Until recently diagnosis has been reliant on detecting virus particles in faecal specimens using electron microscopy. Latex agglutination and enzyme immunoassay kits are among the newer techniques now available as alternatives to electron microscopy. They allow more rapid detection and identification of viruses. Stools can also be examined directly for ova and parasites.

Management

Most acute diarrhoeal episodes are self-limiting. Dehydration is the most common complication of acute diarrhoea and is the main cause of diarrhoea-associated morbidity and mortality. The development of oral rehydration therapy (ORT) has been the major therapeutic advance in the management of acute diarrhoea in recent years. ORT has been shown to be very effective in the treatment of dehydration secondary to diarrhoeal illness. ORT is based on clinical evidence that during acute diarrhoea the bowel can absorb substantial amounts of water and salt taken by mouth provided that the oral solution also contains an actively absorbed organic solute such as glucose or amino acids. Active absorption of these solutes in the small intestine usually continues during diarrhoea, irrespective of its aetiology. Their absorption is linked to that of sodium. When sodium is absorbed, water and electrolytes flow passively in the same direction through intercellular channels to maintain osmotic and ionic equilibrium between the intestinal contents and the child's extracellular fluid. This process is so effective that ORT is considered appropriate for use in rehydration of children with the full spectrum of dehydration.

Where the infant is shocked, intravenous fluids are appropriate. An initial bolus of normal saline 20 ml/kg over 30 minutes will help restore circulating blood volume. Subsequent type and rate of fluid administration depends on the serum sodium level. If there is hypernatraemia, the aim should be to correct the dehydration and the electrolyte disturbance slowly. ORT is safer than intravenous treatment and should be introduced at the earliest opportunity. The child should have frequent clinical and biochemical reviews until the situation is normal.

Traditionally, the outpatient treatment of infants with acute diarrhoea with mild dehydration has consisted of rehydration with clear fluids for 24–48 hours, followed by the introduction of diluted milk or formula, which is slowly increased to normal strength. Dietary restrictions, e.g. lactose-free foods, have also commonly been implemented. However, this practice has little scientific basis and the slow progression to normal diet over several days has serious implications, especially in developing countries, where the nutritional state of the child is often already seriously compromised. We should now aim to achieve rapid rehydration in 4–6 hours with ORT followed by the immediate reintroduction of milk formula. Breastfeeding should continue where possible. Lactose should not be routinely eliminated from the diet. The continuance of loose stools has previously resulted in a reluctance to return children to full diet; these stools should be

Table 2.2 Recommendations for the management of acute diarrhoea

This is divided into three sections (which should be undertaken simultaneously
1. Rehydration
2. Maintenance therapy
3. Replacement of ongoing fluid losses (e.g. diarrhoea)

1. Rehydration

Mildly or moderately dehydrated

a. fluid deficit can be replaced with oral rehydration therapy (ORT) over a 4 hour period.
b. If vomiting, ORT can be given as small frequent volumes.
c. ORT can be used in the presence of hypernatraemia since studies have shown that it is a safe method of normalising serum sodium concentration.
d. If breastfed, do not stop these feeds but give supplemental fluids as ORT.

Severely dehydrated

a. Treat shock if present by restoring circulating volume with normal saline or fresh frozen plasma 20ml/kg IV over 20 minutes. This may need to be repeated.
b. Replace remaining fluid deficit over 12 hours (type of IV fluid will be determined by results of serum sodium, potassium, urea, etc.). Deficit should be corrected slowly if there is hypernatraemia.

2. Maintenance fluids:

a. If still vomiting offer ORT – small amounts frequently (continuing to breastfeed if already breastfed).
b. If not vomiting, continue normal formula feeds and solid feeds. It is not necessary to regrade feeds or to introduce lactose-free diet (unless there is persistently > 1 per cent reducing substances in stools).

3. Replacement of ongoing fluid losses (diarrhoea)

ORT is a rehydration fluid and is not used to stop diarrhoea. Stool consistency should be ignored if child is well. Stool consistency should not influence return to normal diet.

Replace ongoing losses from stools with ORT (= volume of stools passed). Ignore stool consistency if child able to maintain hydration.

ignored if the child can tolerate oral intake. In older children, rice cereal, bananas, potatoes or other foods should be offered shortly after successful rehydration irrespective of the stool consistency or volume (Table 2.2).

The majority of children with acute infectious diarrhoea will not benefit from antimicrobial therapy. In fact, the use of antibiotics in infections like salmonellosis may lead to a prolonged carrier state and an increased risk of bacteriological and symptomatic relapse. Occasionally antibiotics have a role: in patients with certain bacterial and protozoal infections e.g. *Clostridium difficile* (vancomycin, metronidazole), shigella (amoxycillin, trimethoprim-sulphamethoxazone), yersinia (trimethoprim-sulphamethoxazone, chloramphenicol), *Vibrio cholerae* (tetracycline for children over 9 years of age) and *Giardia lamblia* (metronidazole). Currently no antimicrobial agents are effective in the treatment of gastroenteritis caused by viral enteropathogens.

Antidiarrhoeal medications are contraindicated in the management of acute diarrhoea. The principal agents that are used are adsorbants and opiates. Adsorbant preparations used include pectin, kaolin, charcoal and methylcellulose. Their mechanism of action is unclear and their efficacy in treating acute diarrhoea has never been proven. The mechanism of action of opiates is probably to diminish propulsive activity in the intestine. The commonly used opiates in diarrhoea are loperamide, diphenoxylate and codeine. The major concerns in using these agents have been the possibility that they may prolong the intestinal infections by reducing the ability of the gastrointestinal tract to clear the organism, the potential for drug toxicity and masking of symptoms.

Key points

- Oral rehydration solutions are for *re*hydration of *de*hydrated children.
- Treat the child, not the stools.
- Continue feeds unless vomiting is severe.
- Lactose intolerance is rare, and usually transient.
- Intravenous fluids are rarely necessary.
- Antidiarrhoeal drugs should not be used.

Useful literature

- *Treatment of infants with acute diarrhoea: what's recommended and what's practised*, J. Bezerra, T. Stathos, B. Duncan, J. Gaines and J. Udall (*Pediatrics*, vol. 90, pp. 1–4, 1992)
- Dietary management of acute childhood diarrhoea: optimal timing of feeding and appropriate use of milks and mixed diets, K. Brown (*Journal of pediatrics*, vol. 118, pp. S592–8, 1991)
- Therapy for acute infectious diarrhoea in children, L. Pickering (*Journal of pediatrics*, vol. 118, pp. S118-28, 1991)
- *Paediatric gastrointestinal disease*, W. A. Walker, P. Durie, J. Hamilton, J. Walker-Smith and J. Watkins (B.C. Decker Inc, 1991)

3 Acute vomiting

Background

True vomiting occurs as a result of stimulation of a centre in the medulla. It commences with nausea, excessive salivation, pallor and sweating. The stomach is divided by a contraction band at the region of the incisura, a deep inspiration is taken and then, with a strong contraction of the diaphragm and the abdominal muscles, the gastric contents are expelled upwards.

Vomiting is a common symptom in childhood, and children are far more likely to vomit with any given illness than adults. The differential diagnosis of vomiting shows considerable variation with age and it is best to consider vomiting in infancy and childhood separately. The major causes of vomiting in infancy can be broadly categorised into 'normal vomiting', 'sick vomiting' associated with infection or a serious metabolic disturbance, and finally 'mechanical vomiting' associated with anatomical problems such as hiatus hernia and pyloric stenosis (Fig. 3.1). In childhood the major causes of vomiting can be broadly categorised as 'intestinal' and 'cerebral' (Fig. 3.2). As with most clinical presentations, careful history and examination will provide the most useful diagnostic information.

History

Elicit as much detail as possible about the pattern of vomiting. When did it all start? How often is it happening? How much comes up at a time and what colour is it? When children vomit, the initial burst often

INFANCY

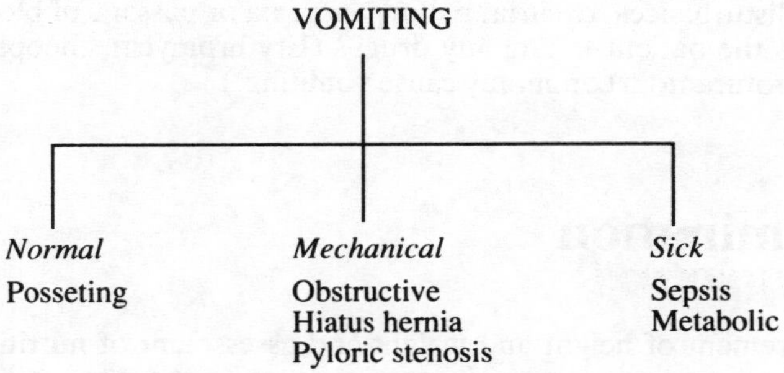

Fig. 3.1 Diagnostic pathway for vomiting in infants. There may be overlap between categories, e.g. shock with obstruction.

CHILDHOOD

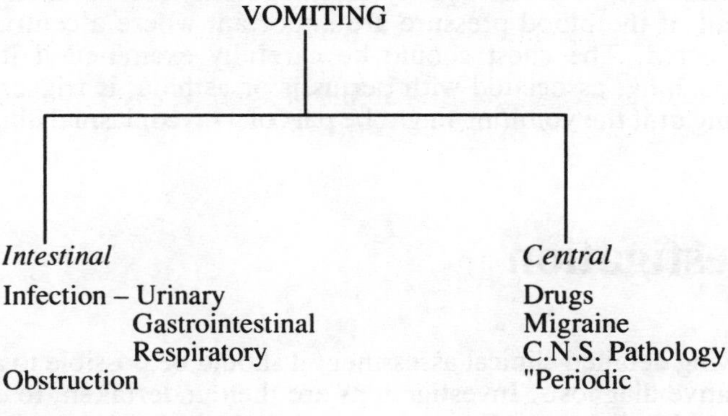

Fig. 3.2 Diagnostic pathway for vomiting in children

contains food or clear secretions from the stomach; later bursts may contain bile-stained fluid from the duodenum; later still, dark brown, 'cola' coloured fluid may be thrown up from the lower small bowel.

Enquire as to precipatory, relieving or aggravatory factors. Is it worsening or improving? Seek relevant associated symptoms such as fever, pain, constipation, diarrhoea, abdominal distension, headache, visual disturbances, dysuria, pallor, anorexia or passage of blood rectally. Is the patient taking any drugs? (Erythromycin, theophyllines and nitrofurantoin commonly cause vomiting.)

Examination

Measurement of height and weight and assessment of nutrition and hydration are mandatory. Inspect the conjunctiva for pallor and jaundice. Smelling the patient's breath may indicate the presence of ketosis or metabolic problems. Where vomitus is available, inspect this.

Pay special attention to abdominal and nervous system examination. Inspect the abdomen for any signs of distension, for movement with respiration and, in small infants, for visible peristalsis in the left upper quandrant and also for visible bowel loops. Palpate specifically for the present of a pyloric tumour or an intussusception in infancy and also look for tenderness suggestive of appendicitis. Tender hepatomegaly will indicate hepatitis. Bowel sounds may be highpitched in the presence of intestinal obstruction or markedly increased where there is gastroenteritis.

Examination of the nervous system, especially the fundi, and measurement of the blood pressure are important where a central cause is suspected. The chest should be carefully examined if it is felt that coughing, associated with pertussis or asthma, is triggering the vomiting or if the vomiting might be part of a mycoplasmal illness.

Investigation

Following detailed clinical assessment it should be possible to achieve a tentative diagnosis. Investigations are then undertaken, to confirm or reject this diagnosis. Investigations are considered in the context of the differential diagnosis which is outlined below.

Infancy (Fig. 3.1)

1. Normal

All babies vomit to some extent. This is sometimes referred to as posseting and probably reflects mild gastro-oesphageal reflux which can be demonstrated in most healthy infants. These children thrive normally and are not distressed by the vomiting, which is a social inconvenience rather than a medical problem. The term 'towel baby' is a useful description – parents bring a towel everywhere to mop up the constant vomits.

2. Sick

Infants with infectious, metabolic and cerebral problems would be included in this category. Patients look unwell and have additional symptoms and signs. Vomiting is a non-specific symptom of meningitis, urinary infection and septicaemia. Coughing, especially that associated with pertussis, often triggers vomiting. Though gastroenteritis is uncommon in early infancy, vomiting may be the first symptom. In the newborn, especially the premature infant, necrotising enterocolitis is a possibility – particularly if the stools are abnormal.

Children with inborn errors of metabolism usually develop symptoms after the ingestion of milk feeds. The child may also be lethargic, anorexic, irritable, tachypnoeic or jaundiced. An unusual smell may be noted. Onset of symptoms may be delayed beyond the first month in cases of partial enzyme deficiency, the disease being unmasked by intercurrent illness. This is a particular problem with maple syrup urine disease, organic acidurias and urea cycle defects.

Raised intracranial pressure may cause vomiting and irritability in infancy. The non-rigid skull of an infant may expand slowly to accommodate gradual onset hydrocephalus with few symptoms, but acute encephalopathies are symptomatic. Meningitis, encephalitis, intracranial haemorrhage and cerebral oedema present with irritability, vomiting, impaired consciousness and seizures. Reye's syndrome of cerebral oedema and fatty liver may be due to a variety of metabolic problems or aspirin ingestion. It typically presents with hypoglycaemia, hepatomegaly and cerebral symptoms including vomiting.

In the infant presenting with 'sick' vomiting, urgent investigation should be undertaken to exclude sepsis and metabolic problems. A 'septic screen' of blood, urine and CSF culture with chest X-ray and white cell count is indicated. Measurement of the blood sugar, urea, electrolytes, liver function tests and blood gas provides a useful initial 'metabolic screen'. Urine should be collected and quickly frozen if an inborn error of metabolism is suspected.

3. Mechanical

This category would include obstruction, pyloric stenosis and severe gastro-oesophageal reflux (GOR).

Congenital intestinal obstruction usually presents in the newborn. Polyhydramnios is usually present and the anatomical diagnosis may be demonstrated by obstetric ultrasound. Bilious vomiting *in utero* may be misinterpreted as meconium passage. The triad of bilious vomiting, abdominal distension and constipation suggests obstruction.

In 'high' obstruction, such as duodenal atresia, distension may not be prominent and meconium can be passed normally. The large distended stomach may accommodate several feeds, so that presentation may be delayed for two to three days. Plain abdominal X-rays are usually adequate for diagnosis and management is surgical. Nasogastric suction and intravenous fluid replacement should be undertaken whilst awaiting surgery.

Malrotation, leading to midgut volvulus, may not present until the infant is several days or months of age. The condition is an emergency, since the bowel will rapidly become devitalised. Presentation is usually with symptoms of obstruction and intestinal ischaemia or infarction. Diagnosis is by a combination of plain X-ray and barium enema or laparotomy. Inguinal or femoral hernia may present with gut obstruction.

Intussusception typically presents in the infant between six and nine months of age. It causes episodes of severe colicky pain. Parents will note paroxysms of pain and pallor, with flexion of the legs. Vomiting and the passage of bloodstained stool follow. Examination of the child when relaxed reveals a palpable, sausage-shaped mass. In cases of doubt, a barium enema is diagnostic and may be therapeutic where paediatric radiological expertise is available. Ultrasound is also useful diagnostically. Intravenous fluid is needed to correct shock due to third space fluid loss, before proceeding to therapeutic radiology or surgery.

Gastro-oesophageal reflux usually presents with a history of chronic vomiting. Where the child is distressed or develops symptoms that suggest oesophagitis, e.g. blood in the vomitus, investigation by means of barium contrast and/or endoscopy is indicated. The management remains controversial. There is a strong natural tendency for symptoms to resolve with time. Where oesophagitis and particularly a partial thoracic stomach is present, long term antiacid treatment is necessary and surgery may warrant consideration.

Pyloric stenosis usually presents in the first month of life with vomiting, which is projectile. The child will usually feed well, but fails to thrive. Where symptoms have been present for some days there will usually be a metabolic upset, loss of hydrochloric acid from the stomach causing a hypochloraemic alkalosis. The diagnosis can usually be made clinically and management is surgical. Ultrasound and barium studies may have a role in diagnosis of atypical cases.

Childhood (Fig. 3.2)

1. Intestinal

Vomiting most commonly occurs as part of gastroenteritis. Vomiting and abdominal pain may precede diarrhoea.

Intestinal obstruction or acute surgical emergencies may also present with vomiting but will usually have other symptoms to suggest the diagnosis. Gastritis due to *Helicobacter pylori* may also present with vomiting which can be chronic. Diagnosis is difficult and may require endoscopy and biopsy. The value of antibody assays in diagnosis is being assessed. Infectious hepatitis may cause nausea and vomiting early in the illness before jaundice is clearly evident. Liver enzymes are elevated and serology will give a more precise diagnosis of A, B or C. Management is supportive. Tonsillitis and otitis media may also cause vomiting.

2. Cerebral

Raised intracranial pressure, though rare, may present with vomiting. There are usually other symptoms and signs such as headache, visual disturbance, neurological dysfunction or hypertension or papilloedema. CT scan is indicated.

Migraine is a prominent cause of vomiting in children. The presence of a typical aura and headache along with a family history usually suggest the diagnosis. 'Abdominal migraine' is seen in a number of children with migraine where vomiting and abdominal pain are the principal symptoms. There is an overlap between this condition and non-specific recurrent abdominal pain which occurs in approximately 10 per cent of children and is associated with vomiting in approximately a quarter. The diagnosis is clinical.

Certain drugs can cause vomiting and mediate their effect centrally. These include many of the cytotoxic chemotherapeutic agents and more commonly used drugs such as theophylline and erythromycin. These latter drugs also interact so that the addition of erythromycin to a patient stable on theophylline will usually cause vomiting.

As in infancy, vomiting may be a symptom of serious infection such as meningitis or part of a generalised infectious or metabolic process.

Severe coughing, particularly that associated with pertussis, asthma or mycoplasma infection, may also give rise to vomiting.

Key points

- Children vomit more readily than adults.
- Bilious vomiting in the in the newborn is caused by intestinal obstruction until proven otherwise
- Beware the lethargic infant who vomits – suspect sepsis or metabolic problems
- The triad of early morning headache, vomiting and visual disturbance suggests raised intracranial pressure.
- Nausea and vomiting often precede jaundice in cases of infectious hepatitis.
- Erythromycin, nitrofurantoin and theophylline cause vomiting.

4 Bleeding and bruising

Introduction

Bruising is a very common problem in childhood and surveys of normal children have shown that over one third of all children will have some evidence of minor injury – usually bruises – when carefully examined. The incidence of minor bruising is low during infancy and then rises steadily to the age of three when around 60 per cent of children will have some bruising. Bruising due to non-accidental injury is much less common and tends to have a distribution unrelated to the developmental age of the child. Bruising and bleeding may be caused by various types of bleeding diatheses and the differential diagnosis can often be narrowed down by careful attention to the clinical presentation.

Evaluation

History

There may be great anxiety associated with the presentation of bleeding and bruising when this is unrelated to injury. The history is of critical importance. When non-accidental injury is suspected details of the event should be recorded verbatim. In the past history, determine whether or not there was any significant bleeding after dental extraction, tonsillectomy or circumcision. Dental extraction, in particular, is a solid challenge to haemostasis and is likely to unmask any latent bleeding diathesis. The time of onset of bleeding or bruising should be noted, many disorders of coagulation may not present until the baby starts to become mobile. The family history is important in many coagulation and vascular disorders and a detailed pedigree should be drawn if there is any suspicion of an inherited disorder.

Differential diagnosis

Generalised bleeding and bruising may be due to either a bleeding tendency or trauma. 'Single-site' bleeding is most commonly due to local pathology, e.g. melaena in Meckel's diverticulum and will not be considered further. Haemostasis may be compromised by problems caused by vascular disorders, thrombocytopenia or coagulation deficiencies. Disorders of platelet function and circulating anticoagulants may also occur but they are very rare.

Bleeding and bruising due to trauma in children are usually accidental but be aware that non-accidental injury is always a possibility and pay careful attention to accurate recording of the type and distribution of the bruising. Bruising due to vascular disorders may be either congenital, such as Ehlers–Danlos syndrome, or acquired, such as vasculitis due to Henoch–Schonlein purpura or acute meningococcaemia. Thrombocytopenia may be due to reduced production of platelets as in congenital or acquired disorders of the bone marrow. Hypersplenism or platelet antibodies may cause thrombocytopenia due to increased destruction. Coagulation disorders may be inherited, as for instance in haemophilia and Christmas disease, or acquired as in vitamin K deficiency and disseminated intravascular coagulation.

Clinical examination

Most children will not be acutely ill at the time of initial examination, but acute presentations need to be rapidly evaluated and in some cases, e.g. acute meningococcaemia, require emergency treatment. In meningococcal septicaemia the child may often be in early shock – a drowsy child with poor peripheral perfusion, tachycardia and evolving petechiae or purpura should be managed as meningococcaemia until proven otherwise. Most other presentations will be subacute and allow time for careful and detailed examination.

In the first place, establish that the spots are true petechiae or purpura and not erythematous spots or telangiectasiae. This can be simply done by noting the absence of blanching on pressure with petechiae and purpura. Petechiae usually signify disorders of a vascular origin or thrombocytopenia. These disorders may also be associated with purpura. In contrast, coagulation deficiencies tend to present with deeper bruising and haematomata. Petechiae and purpura due to vascular and platelet disorders tend to be associated with spontaneous bleeding, whereas bleeding due to coagulation disorders is often related to minor trauma. The distribution of petechiae is important and when due to vascular or platelet disorders, is usually generalised.

Petechiae due to raised intracapillary pressure are common and tend to occur in the distribution of the superior vena cava. This type of presentation in children is caused by raised venous pressure in situations which provoke a response similar to a prolonged Valsalva manoeuvre. Thus, this pattern of petechiae is seen in whooping cough and used to be relatively common when stomach washouts were the order of the day in the management of acute poisoning. Local 'traumatic' petechiae may be seen after prolonged application of a tourniquet – for example when siting an intravenous line. Purpura associated with vasculitis, such as Henoch–Schonlein

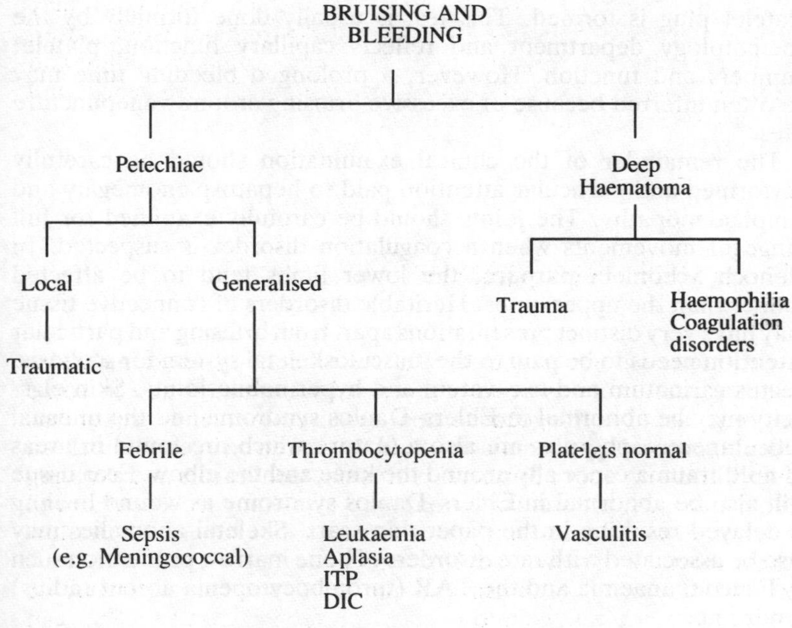

Fig. 4.1 Diagnostic pathway for recent onset bruising and bleeding

purpura, will often have associated inflammation and the purpura may be preceded by an urticarial rash before becoming purpuric after a day or two. Bruising due to injury will tend to have a different distribution depending on whether the cause is accidental or non-accidental.

Bruising in the lower limbs is just as common in accidental and non-accidental injury except in infancy. Bruising in the lumbar region is more common in non-accidental injury and especially in those children less than five years of age. Children of school age may have some lumbar bruising due to injuries at play with other children (see Chapter 6).

Bruising in the region of the head and face is much more common in non-accidental injury in all ages though bruising in this area can be accidental in the toddler age group.

The Hess test can be used to investigate capillary resistance and may be abnormal in children when there is increased capillary fragility due to a vascular disorder or thrombocytopenia. A blood pressure cuff is inflated to the mean blood pressure for five minutes: there should be less than five petechiae in an area of 5 cm in diameter just below the elbow. The bleeding time is a measure of how long it takes to seal a small skin puncture as the platelet plug is formed. This test is usually done formally by the haematology department and reflects capillary function, platelet numbers and function. However, a prolonged bleeding time may be often inferred because of excessive bruising around venepuncture sites.

The remainder of the clinical examination should be carefully performed and particular attention paid to hepatosplenomegaly and lymphadenopathy. The joints should be carefully examined for full range of movements when a coagulation disorder is suspected. In Henoch–Schonlein purpura, the lower limbs tend to be affected sooner than the upper limbs. Heritable disorders of connective tissue may have very distinct presentations apart from bruising and particular attention needs to be paid to the musculoskeletal system for scoliosis, pectus carinatum and excavatum and hypermobile joints. Skin elasticity may be abnormal in Ehlers–Danlos syndrome and the unusual subcutaneous spherules are also a feature which are found in areas of mild trauma especially around the knee and the elbow. Scar tissue will also be abnormal in Ehlers–Danlos syndrome as wound healing is delayed resulting in the paper-thin scars. Skeletal anomalies may also be associated with rare disorders of bone marrow production such as Fanconi anaemia and the TAR (thrombocytopenia absent radius) syndrome.

Investigations

Investigations will be very much determined by the clinical examination. Clearly no special investigations are indicated in accidental bruising and petechiae due to raised intravascular pressure. A coagulation screen and a platelet count are important for medico-legal reasons when non-accidental injury is suspected. Poor sampling technique may affect the platelet count but this is usually detected by the finding of small clots in the sample. There will usually not be spontaneous petechiae unless the platelet count is below 40 000. Most haematology laboratories will have a screening test for the intrinsic and the extrinsic coagulation system. The extrinsic coagulation factors are measured by the prothrombin ratio which reflects the vitamin K dependent liver factors of II, VII, IX and X and a test of the clotting time, such as the kaolin cephalin time, will reflect the factors of the intrinsic coagulation system. More detailed factor analysis can be done when specific deficiencies are suspected.

Thrombocytopenia is most commonly caused by idiopathic thrombocytopenic purpura or an infiltrative disorder of the bone marrow. Bone marrow examination will help to exclude any serious underlying disorder and in some cases bone marrow chromosomes may help establish or qualify the underlying diagnosis.

The bleeding diathesis associated with acute septicaemia will often have complex haematological findings reflecting disseminated intravascular coagulation. There may be thrombocytopenia, deficiency of the labile coagulation factors V and VIII, circulating anticoagulants and raised fibrin degradation products (FDPs).

Management

Toddler bruising only requires reassurance but bruising due to non-accidental injury requires the difficult and prolonged process of accurate documentation, case conferences and possible court proceedings.

The commonest cause of thrombocytopenia in paediatrics is idiopathic thrombocytopenic purpura. Steroids or human immunoglobulin and platelet transfusions are used for those cases at risk of serious bleeding i.e. counts less than 40 000. Thrombocytopenia due to bone marrow infiltration is managed by treating the underlying condition and this may range from combination chemotherapy in acute leukaemia to bone marrow transplantation for aplastic anaemia.

Specific coagulation factor replacement is required in the congenital deficiency disorders such as haemophilia and Christmas disease and increasingly children and parents are becoming more efficient at managing this condition at home.

Prophylactic vitamin K in the newborn has recently become controversial because of a UK study suggesting an association with childhood cancer, although this has not been substantiated in the United States or Sweden. Vitamin K prophylaxis should continue to be given in the newborn and especially to those babies who are breastfed, as late haemorrhagic disease in the newborn with intracranial haemorrhage is commonest in exclusively breastfed babies.

In special situations platelet transfusions may be given but these are rarely indicated unless there is significant bleeding associated with a platelet count less than 10 000. Similarly in the acutely ill child, the management of disseminated intravascular coagulation is essentially that of the underlying disorder but there may be occasions when the coagulation factor replacement may be necessary using fresh plasma or concentrates.

Key points

- Healthy toddlers often have bruises on the forehead, knees, shins and forearms.
- Disorders of clotting factors tend to cause deep haematomata.
- Spontaneous generalised petechiae are usually due to thrombocytopenia.
- Localised petechiae may be caused by transient increased venous pressure, e.g. prolonged coughing, straining or application of a tourniquet.
- Prothrombin time, partial thromboplastin time, bleeding time and platelet count will categorise most bleeding problems.

Useful literature

- Haematologic disorders, P. Lane, R. Nuss and J. Ambruso. In: *Current paediatric diagnosis and treatment*, W. Hathway, W. Hay, J. Groothuis and J. Paisley (eds) (Prentice-Hall, 1993)

5 The collapsed child

The child who arrives in the emergency room looking extremely ill or unconscious may be described as 'collapsed'. This presentation can indicate almost anything. It is helpful to develop a system of management and rapid diagnostic categorisation, as this will assist the efficiency and effectiveness of the response. Where a child has sustained a cardiorespiratory arrest out of hospital, resuscitation attempts should be tempered by the knowledge that the possibility of intact survival is slim. Similarly, where the terminal deterioration is part of a fatal illness, resuscitation may not be appropriate.

Assessment and first aid

Calmly assess along A,B,C lines. If a coherent relative is present try to obtain essential items of history whilst assessing. Don't be 'brave', get senior help and advice quickly.

Airway

Be sure the child is in the lateral position and that the airway is not obstructed. Is the child breathing, is the chest wall moving equally and are there good breath sounds? Is the child pink?

Breathing

Where there is concern regarding breathing, an arterial gas may clarify matters. If the child is obviously in difficulty, bag and mask ventilation or intubation with intermittent positive pressure ventilation may be indicated.

Circulation

Check for circulatory integrity. Monitor the pulse rate and volume, the blood pressure and tissue perfusion (capillary refill time).

Establish vascular access

This may be technically the most difficult part of the procedure. Try to develop a systematic way of looking for 'usable' veins. Inspect the hands, wrists, elbows, ankles, groin, scalp and neck. The choice of access will depend on what is visible and on the skills and preferences of the operator. Where access has not been obtained within a couple of minutes, get a senior colleague. Consideration may be given to a cut-down or to inserting a needle in the bone marrow (tibia) if the child is ill and unconscious. Arterial access is very valuable for monitoring blood gases and blood pressure in acutely ill children. It is perhaps best to place the arterial line when the child has been stabilised in an intensive care setting and after local anaesthesia.

Document the clinical and laboratory status

Treatment, information gathering and monitoring must proceed rapidly together. Monitor the pulse, respiratory rate, blood pressure and temperature. It is particularly valuable to simultaneously measure core and peripheral temperature as an index of perfusion. Pulse oximetry will give a useful guide to oxygen levels, but should not be used to assess ventilation. Blood gases and sugar (stick test) should be measured urgently to assess whether there are respiratory or metabolic problems. Urine flow should be monitored and if necessary, the bladder catheterised. Further essential information is provided by a full blood count, electrolytes, urea, septic screen and chest X-ray.

Specific treatment

This will depend on the cause of the problem. The broad differential will be 1. shock, 2. cardiac, 3. respiratory and 4. cerebral (Fig. 5.1).

Shock

Shock may be due to sepsis, blood loss due to bleeding or sickling, dehydration or metabolic disturbance such as adrenal failure, poisoning, inborn errors of metabolism, diabetes or hypoglycaemia. Management of shock which is causing collapse will require information as to whether the shock is associated with hypovolaemia. Where this distinction is not clinically apparent, measurement of central venous pressure is necessary. Fluid therapy will be influenced by the clinical and biochemical assessments. It should be regulated according to the response of the patient in terms of blood pressure, peripheral perfusion, urine flow and central venous pressure (CVP). Where hypotension persists despite adequate fluid volume, inotropic support in the form of dopamine or dobutamine is required. These agents should always be administered through a central line.

Specific measures to deal with poisoning are best undertaken having consulted with the local poisons unit. An aplastic crisis in sickle cell disease causing profound anaemia may require urgent exchange transfusion. Where sepsis is the cause of shock antibiotics are necessary; a concomitant intravascular coagulation may require treatment with plasma and platelets. The use of steroids and anti-

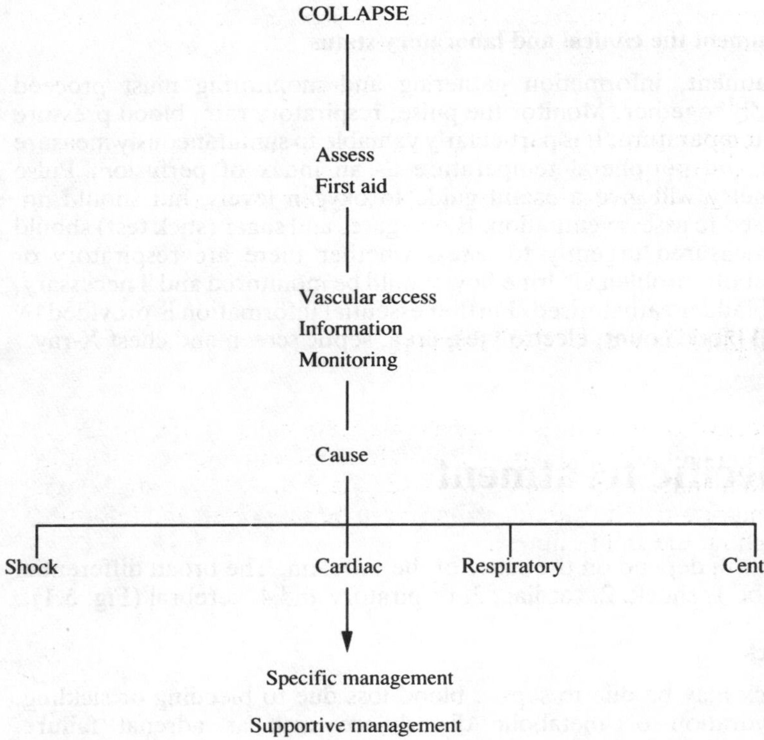

Fig. 5.1 Management and assessment pathway for acute collapse

endotoxin antibodies have been advocated but there is no consensus as to their efficacy.

Cardiac

Cardiac causes of collapse will include acute onset arrhythmia (e.g. supraventricular tachycardia (SVT)), severe infundibular spasm (Fallot's tetralogy) and onset of congestive heart failure. SVT may be managed with immersion in iced water, intravenous adenosine or DC cardioversion. Infundibular spasm is best managed with sedation using morphine and occasionally propranolol. Congestive heart failure will require standard treatment with oxygen and diuretics and investigation to define the cause.

Acute respiratory failure

Acute respiratory failure may be associated with pneumothorax, asthma, inhaled foreign body or infection. Specific treatment is straightforward, respiratory failure will need to be managed conventionally with oxygen and/or positive pressure ventilation.

Cerebral

Neurological causes of acute collapse are usually associated with prolonged fitting. Management will involve terminating the seizure and treating any infection or raised intracranial pressure.

Supportive treatment

Irrespective of the cause of the child's acute collapse there may be complicating multi-organ problems. These require ongoing monitoring and management. The need for adequate analgesia throughout is very important. The parents will need to be supported and informed throughout the child's illness.

Key points

- Cardiac arrest in children most commonly occurs as a result of respiratory failure or shock! Asystole (rather than ventricular fibrillation) is usual.
- Don't be 'brave' – get senior help and advice.
- Properly used bag and mask will provide adequate ventilation in the absence of airway obstruction. Valuable time may be wasted attempting intubation.
- Urgent access to the circulation may be obtained using a wide gauge needle in the tibial marrow.
- The outcome for unwitnessed cardiac arrest is very poor.

Useful literature

- *Essentials of pediatric intensive care manual*, Toro-Figueroa, H. Levin and F. Morriss. (Quality Medical Publishing, 1992)
- *Advanced paediatric life support.* Advanced life support group, British Medical Journal Publishing Group, London, 1993.

6 Child abuse

Introduction

While child abuse is not a modern phenomenon, it was not until 1962 that Henry Kempe forced reluctant professionals to acknowledge that the problem exists and to develop strategies to deal with it, when he used the term 'Battered baby syndrome'. The term child abuse has expanded to include the following forms of ill treatment:

1. Physical injury
2. Emotional abuse and failure to thrive
3. Neglect
4. Poisoning
5. Child sexual abuse.

The prevalence of child abuse is difficult to determine accurately, most statistics being underestimates. Current estimates of prevalence of child abuse in Western societies range between 10–20 cases per 1000 live births.

Physical abuse

The majority of physically abused children are less than two years of age. Males are at a greater risk. The abused child may have a chronic illness or handicap, being different from his siblings. The child may be hyperactive and difficult to control or may have been the result of an unwanted pregnancy. The abusive parents are more likely to have been abused themselves as children and to have a psychiatric disorder. The family background is often chaotic, abuse being more common in lower socioeconomic groups, single parent families and in the presence of marital disharmony.

The injuries inflicted vary in severity, some leading to death or permanent disabilities. When a dead child is brought into hospital, it is important to examine the body carefully to exclude signs of bruising, injury or neglect. A small proportion of cases of sudden infant death syndrome have been attributed to suffocation. Children who die as a result of abuse may have presented with recurring minor injuries in the past, such minor injuries representing the parents 'cry for help'.

Intracranial injuries may occur as a result of a direct blow to the head or as a result of violent shaking. In the former, skull fractures commonly involve the parietal bone. The fractures tend to be multiple and irregular. There may be an underlying subdural haematoma or cerebral oedema. Shake injuries occur in children less than 2 years of age. In this form of injury the child is shaken violently by the parent causing both intracranial and intraocular bleeds. There are often grasp marks on the upper arms or trunk. The child may present with unexplained loss of consciousness and in all such cases examination of the fundi to exclude intraocular bleeds is mandatory. The outlook for children with shake injuries is poor.

Table 6.1 Child abuse

Clinical Examination
Bruises
Any bruises on a baby less than one year of age
Bruising from human bites
Black eyes
Bruising of ear and scalp
Petechial haemorrhages
Finger and thumb marks
Fractures
Any in the first year
Burns
Circular and discrete
Immersion

Bruising particularly affects the head and face, where the soft tissues are injured. The pinnae, cheeks and mouth are not normally bruised when an accidental injury occurs. The frenulum may be torn as a result of an upward blow to the mouth. Bruises may be of differing ages. The pattern of bruising may indicate the weapon used such as a hand, rod, slipper or belt. Pinching causes a typical bruise pattern. Human bites can be distinguished from animal bites by the regular oval pattern of the abrasion from a human bite as opposed to irregular jagged abrasion associated with animal bites.

Bruising as a result of play or injury is uncommon in children in their first year of life. In this age group any bruising should be treated with suspicion. In all cases where child abuse is suspected, the pattern of bruising must be carefully documented, photographed and a bleeding disorder excluded by performing clotting studies. The parents' explanation for the injury may be inadequate or inconsistent. Particular attention should be paid to any discrepancy between the given story and the child's motor developmental age. Six-week-old infants do not roll off their cots on to the floor. As with the pattern of bruising, the parents' history must be carefully recorded.

Fractures as a result of abuse tend to be multiple and may be of differing ages. Fractures under one year of age are particularly significant. A full skeletal survey should be performed in all cases of suspected physical abuse to detect fractures of differing ages at varying stages of healing. Marked periosteal reaction may be present. In cases of doubt, X-rays should be repeated after a two week interval or isotope bone scans can be performed. Avulsion fractures of the growing end of long bones, multiple epiphyseal fractures, posterior rib fractures and spiral fractures of the long bones due to twist injury are all suggestive of abuse. As in other forms of physical abuse, there may be a delay of several days between the onset of the injury and the seeking of appropriate treatment.

Burns usually occur by accident, but the pattern of burn may be suggestive of abuse. Multiple circular discrete burns with blistering and secondary infection indicate cigarette burns, where the cigarette has been held against the skin for several seconds. This contrasts with accidental cigarette burns where contact is brief causing minimal erythema. Scalding may involve immersion with scalds affecting both hands or feet, extending to the level of the ankles or wrists. If the child is placed in a scalding hot bath, the buttocks will also be involved. The pattern of the burn may indicate whether there has been deliberate contact with a hot plate, poker or bar of an electric fire.

Awareness of conditions that mimic abusive injuries is important so that misdiagnosis is avoided. These include accidental injuries, abnormal bone fragility as in osteogenesis imperfecta or pathological fractures associated with malignancy. Bleeding disorders must be excluded. Neurological conditions associated with sensory loss may give rise to severe accidental injury or burns. Dermatological disorders may present with scarring or blistering. The Mongolian blue spot should not be mistaken for bruising. Periosteal reaction may be seen in scurvy or congenital syphilis.

Table 6.2 Assessment

Detailed history:	1. Explanation 2. Previous incidents 3. Siblings
Examination:	1. Fully undressed 2. Photograph 3. Centile chart
Investigation:	1. Clotting studies 2. Skeletal survey

Emotional abuse and failure to thrive

Emotional abuse occurs when there is an absence of normal parental care with failure to show the expected concern and love for the child. It occurs in all social backgrounds and it is extremely difficult to detect. It may be passive, involving such practices as leaving a child unattended for long periods, not showing affection or failing to stimulate and encourage a child when appropriate. Active abuse includes threatening the child repeatedly, limiting peer contact and play experiences by confining the child to a limited space such as a cupboard or cellar, and the undermining of self-esteem by constant criticism.

Failure to thrive is due to non-organic causes in 50 per cent of cases, this occurring most commonly in lower socioeconomic groups. The family is often dysfunctional with many background problems, such as marital disharmony, drug abuse, psychiatric illness and unemployment. The child may have an underlying chronic illness or handicap. Such a child may be a scapegoat within the family, his siblings being given appropriate care and nutrition. Both the height and weight may be below the third centile, with abnormal growth velocity.

There may be associated emotional disturbances, the child being withdrawn, uncommunicative and fearful. Following provision of a caring environment, including a period of hospitalisation, there is characteristically a period of rapid increase in height and weight towards normal centiles, although eventual growth potential may be limited. When a child thrives normally in hospital, but fails to do so when returned home, underlying abuse must be seriously considered.

Neglect

There is a considerable overlap between neglect, emotional abuse and non-organic failure to thrive. Neglected children may be left unattended for long periods, putting them at risk of injury or death as a result of home accidents. They may not be provided with adequate nutrition, shelter, protection from injury or medical care. Severely neglected children are pale, sad and apathetic. The hair may be sparse and dry. The skin is often mottled with acrocyanosis. In neglected infants nappy rashes may be untreated, clothing poor and hygiene minimal. The neglecting parents may have attained poor educational standards, with resulting inadequate personal and financial resources.

Poisoning

Poisoning should be considered when a child presents with episodes of unexplained illness, associated with unusual biochemical disturbances, drowsiness and loss of consciousness. Episodes may be repetitive and in such circumstances a toxicology screen should be performed. Because of the abnormal biochemical profile, a metabolic disorder may be suspected, especially when associated with underlying neurological symptoms such as convulsion or coma.

Poisoning may be part of the fabrication of illness seen in Munchausen's syndrome by proxy. In a typical case a child presents with persistent or recurring illness that cannot be explained. There is a discrepancy between clinical findings and the history. The symptoms and signs do not make clinical sense. The diagnosis considered is usually that of a rare disorder and attempts at treatment are unsuccessful. Symptoms and signs do not occur in the absence of the parent, usually the mother. It is rarely seen in children older than 6 years.

Child sexual abuse

Kempe in 1978 defined child sexual abuse as 'the involvement of dependent, developmentally immature children and adolescents in sexual activities that they do not fully comprehend, to which they are unable to give informed consent, or that violate the social taboos or family role'. The act of abuse may vary from involvement in prostitution, pornographic pictures or films, inappropriate touching and attempted or actual genital, oral or anal penetration.

Its prevalence is as common as all other forms of abuse. The abuser is more likely to be male and a family member, relative or carer. As in physical abuse, abusers are more likely to have been sexually abused in their own childhood.

Awareness that a child is being sexually abused may occur when a child discloses the fact to a carer. In these circumstances any details the child gives must be accurately recorded. The child should be believed and reassured that it is safe and correct to give details of the abusive acts, as they will usually have been threatened by the abuser that there will be serious consequences for the child or family if the abuse is revealed. Children should also be guaranteed protection and provided with strategies to ensure that abuse will not recur.

Table 6.3 Child sexual abuse – initial responses

Stay calm.
Listen carefully.
Don't make promises of complete confidentiality.
Consult with colleagues.
Inform the appropriate Child Protection Agency.

In the absence of a statement from the child, child sexual abuse may be suspected as a result of the child's inappropriate sexual knowledge or sexualised behaviour. Emotional disturbance may be a presenting feature, although such problems as enuresis, anorexia and truancy, are not specific to child sexual abuse. As a consequence of physical injury there may be genital or anal discharge, irritation or bleeding. Abnormal physical signs are present in only 25 per cent of abused children, their absence therefore not excluding the possibility that child sexual abuse has taken place.

Having interviewed the child, a physical examination is required.

This should only be carried out by a doctor who is familiar with normal and abnormal paediatric genital anatomy. Multiple physical examinations must be avoided. Where an acute abusive incident has occurred, full forensic examination is required with samples being taken as appropriate to local circumstances. In the majority of cases abuse has been chronic so that one can plan the examination at some time when an expert is available.

The planned examination should take place in the presence of a parent or carer. Before the examination is performed a full menstrual history and history of any accidents in the genital or anal areas is obtained. The child's demeanour, growth, pubertal status and development should be noted. In post-pubertal girls the possibility of pregnancy should be considered. The presence of bruising, bite marks or burns in the genital and anal area are recorded. Scarring or abrasions may be seen in the vaginal introitus. Detection is indicative of actual or attempted penetrative sexual abuse. Chronic anal abuse may give rise to anal dilatation, fissures or scarring. Where a vaginal or anal discharge is present swabs should be taken to detect sexually transmitted disease.

The results of the examination must be conveyed to the child and his or her parents or guardians. The physical examination is only a part of the overall assessment of child sexual abuse as abnormal physical signs are rarely unequivocally diagnostic of child sexual abuse. Exceptions are the detection of semen or blood of a different group to that of the child on examination.

Management of the abused child

Once suspected, the protection of the abused child is a priority. In most cases it is advisable to remove the child from the abusive environment. This prevents further abuse from occurring and facilitates further assessment. Many children are admitted to hospital for this purpose. In hospital the pattern of abuse is documented, appropriate investigation is performed and treatment given. The paediatrician, should inform the appropriate child protection agency. He should also meet with the parents, in the presence of the hospital or community social worker, to inform them of the diagnosis and to obtain further information as to the origin of the injuries.

A multidisciplinary case conference must be held at which information about the child's injuries, the child's background and family circumstances are exchanged with those who are already involved with the family. This may include the general practitioner, public health visitor, police and teacher. Representatives of the Child Protection Agency are also present. Having discussed the injuries and background a decision is made as to what action should be taken with particular reference to child protection issues. The decision is conveyed to the parents and the child.

Should the parents refuse to allow their child to be admitted for a period of assessment or attempt to remove their child before investigations are completed, a Place of Safety Order should be sought. This is granted by a court on application and lasts for a fixed period. Having completed investigations, a decision may be made by the case conference:

- To allow the child home as abuse wasn't confirmed;
- To allow the child home but to apply to the court for a supervision order. This obliges the parents to allow members of the Child Protection Agency to have access to the home to supervise the child's progress. It also may oblige them to bring the child for a particular course of therapy;
- Where the child is considered to be at grave risk, a Care Order is applied for in the juvenile courts. If granted, the care of the child passes from the parents to the Child Protection Agency.

The management of child sexual abuse should never be the responsibility of one person alone. If a doctor suspects abuse, he should consult colleagues and the local Child Protection Agency for advice. The assessment of child sexual abuse is particularly difficult and in most areas, special teams have been established for this purpose to whom the referral should be made. Where sexual abuse is suspected, it is more appropriate that the abuser, if known, leaves home, rather than the child. Hospital admission for further assessment is, in most cases, inappropriate.

When abuse has occurred, particularly if it has been chronic, the child may have suffered considerable psychological damage. In these circumstances, considerations must be given not only to the protection of the child from further abuse but also to providing psychiatric treatment to reverse any damage. It can no longer be considered adequate simply to remove the child from an abusing environment or to remove the abuser from home. Long-term intervention strategies are required to prevent the abused children becoming abusers themselves when they reach adulthood.

Key points

- When child abuse is suspected – always inform a senior colleague.
- Most 'serious' physical abuse is perpetrated on infants and toddlers.
- Facial and truncal bruising is unusual in children – beware.
- If sexual abuse is suspected – ensure that only one examination is performed.
- Record exactly what is said, and by whom.

7 Cough

Cough is a common symptom in clinical practice. It has two very important physiological functions, namely to protect the airway from aspiration and to expel secretions and exudate from the lower respiratory tract. In normal circumstances cilial activity is sufficient to clear the airways of secretions but when secretions are excessive, such as in asthma, or cilial activity is damaged, such as in acute infection, effective coughing is essential. It is useful at the outset to distinguish the acute development of a cough in a previously well child from an exacerbation of a chronic cough (Fig. 7.1).

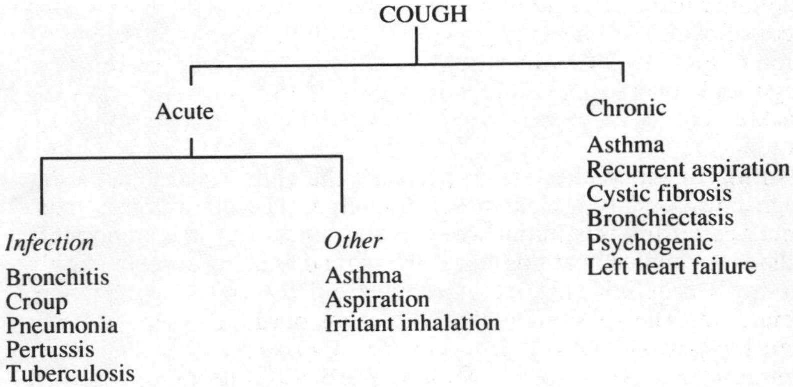

Fig. 7.1 Diagnostic pathway for cough

Acute cough

Probably the commonest cause of acute cough is viral bronchitis, a frequent condition in young children. There may be associated upper respiratory tract symptoms suggestive of a viral aetiology, e.g. rhinorrhoea. Attacks are more common during the winter months and the symptoms usually last for 7–10 days. Persistence of symptoms for longer than two weeks suggests a complication such as a superimposed bacterial infection or segmental collapse. It can be difficult to distinguish recurrent acute viral bronchitis from infrequent episodic asthma and a trial of bronchodilator therapy is appropriate if there is any doubt.

A harsh barking cough in association with hoarseness and stridor occurs in 'croup'. Most cases are viral in origin (acute laryngotracheobronchitis) and typically the child has coryzal symptoms for a couple of days prior to the onset of the croup. Fever is common but usually mild. A small proportion of cases are recurrent and not associated with respiratory infection. Typically the child wakes during the night with croup having been perfectly well on going to bed. The aetiology of this 'spasmodic' croup is unclear but there is some evidence that it has an allergic basis and may evolve to typical asthma.

Cough may not be a prominent feature of pneumonia, particularly in the early stages. In bacterial pneumonia in infancy, symptoms at the onset are often non-specific, such as vomiting and irritability before cough and respiratory distress develop. In older children chest and abdominal pains are common due to pleuritic involvement and signs of consolidation are usually present. In viral pneumonias the constitutional upset and breathlessness are usually more marked than the cough and specific signs on examination of the chest are variable. Crackles are usually present but signs of lobar consolidation are unusual.

During the coryzal phase of pertussis the child usually has a dry cough and possibly a clear nasal discharge. The condition is most infectious during this initial week of the illness but it is impossible to diagnose clinically at this stage, the diagnosis being suspected only if there is a definite history of contact and the child has not been immunised. The spasmodic phase develops during the second week when the paroxysmal cough, occurring in spasms and ending in an inspiratory whoop, is usually present. Paroxysms are more common at night and are frequently followed by vomiting. The whoop is often absent in young infants who may develop apnoeic spells following a paroxysm. Despite the severity of the cough, systemic upset is not prominent and the lungs are usually clear.

Night sweats, weight loss and poor social circumstances raise the possibility of tuberculosis in a child who presents with a cough. In a child with cough due to irritant gas inhalation, there is usually a history of exposure to the toxic fumes. Onset of coughing following a choking spell or vomit is suggestive of aspiration.

Chronic cough

Asthma is the commonest cause of chronic cough in childhood affecting at least 10 per cent of all children. Seasonal variations, nocturnal exacerbations, precipitation by exercise, upper respiratory tract infection and emotional upset support the diagnosis as does the presence of another atopic condition in the child or a positive family history of atopy. The majority of children with an exacerbation of asthma will have an associated wheeze.

Chronic cough associated with vomiting is suggestive of recurrent aspiration secondary to gastro-oesophageal reflux. If the cough has been present since birth and the X-ray appearances are suggestive of recurrent aspiration the possibility of an H-type tracheo-oesophageal fistula arises.

Cystic fibrosis may present with cough but usually other features of the condition are also present such as failure to thrive, chronic diarrhoea and finger clubbing. The development of a chronic cough following a lower respiratory tract infection should raise the possibility of bronchiectasis.

Psychogenic coughing is also a possibility, in which case there will be no evidence of underlying organic disease and the cough will not occur during sleep. A persistent dry cough is common in left ventricular failure and may be the presenting symptom in children with cardiomyopathy. Clinical examination of the cardiovascular system will make the diagnosis clear in such cases.

Investigations (Table 7.1)

In many cases the diagnosis is obvious following a clinical assessment and investigations are unnecessary. A chest X-ray is warranted if pneumonia is suspected or the cough is long-standing. The pattern of radiological change may suggest a specific diagnosis, e.g. inflammatory changes in both lower lobes and sometimes the right upper lobe may occur with recurrent aspiration. When infection is suspected an attempt should be made to obtain sputum for culture. The majority of young children swallow sputum but a sample can often be obtained by positioning the child over a chair and getting them to cough. Blood eosinophilia or raised IgE levels may suggest asthma and marked lymphocytosis usually occurs in the early stages of pertussis. In the majority of cases the blood count is not helpful.

Table 7.1 Cough investigations

Common	Chest X-ray Sputum culture Differential WCC Pulmonary function tests Sweat test Immunoglobulins Mantoux
Occasional	Bronchoscopy Oesophageal pH monitoring Barium swallow Detailed immunological work-up including HIV Chest CT Ciliary analysis

Pulmonary function tests before and after bronchodilator therapy may confirm a diagnosis of asthma in older children. A sweat test and immunoglobulin levels are indicated if the child is failing to thrive in association with recurrent chest infections. A Mantoux test should be performed if there is any suspicion of tuberculosis.

A number of other investigations may occasionally be necessary. If foreign body inhalation is strongly suspected a bronchoscopy is indicated. Gastro-oesophageal reflux is best evaluated by oesophageal pH monitoring. A barium swallow may also be helpful and it should be performed with the patient prone if H-type tracheo-oesophageal fistula is suspected. Detailed immunological investigations should be performed if the cough is associated with recurrent severe infections involving the skin and gastrointestinal tract as well as the chest. In such circumstances the possibility of HIV should also be considered. Chest CT scanning is useful in diagnosing and assessing the extent of bronchiectasis and has largely replaced bronchography. The possibility of ciliary dyskinesia is raised if a child with bronchiectasis has had a chronic cough with nasal stuffiness dating from the neonatal period. The diagnosis is made by looking for characteristic changes in the cilia from nasal brushings. A proportion of such patients will have dextrocardia in which case the diagnosis is Kartagener's syndrome.

Treatment

Cough is a symptom rather than a diagnosis and its treatment is more likely to be effective if it is directed at the underlying cause rather than simply using a cough suppressant. Inhaled bronchodilator therapy through an appropriate device with or without prophylactic treatment is required if the cough is asthmatic in origin. Antibiotic treatment is prescribed if the cough is due to a bacterial infection although the majority of infective cases have a viral aetiology. Gastro-oesophageal reflux is treated medically in the first instance; a small proportion of cases require Nissen's fundoplication.

Antitussives have a very limited role in the management of children. Cough suppressants are not recommended, and 'expectorants' are of no value.

Key points

- Asthma is the most common cause of chronic or recurrent cough.
- Paroxysomal cough with vomiting is usually due to pertussis.
- Psychogenic cough disappears during sleep.
- Mucolytics, expectorants and cough suppressants are rarely useful.

Useful literature

- *Respiratory illness in children*, 3rd edition, P. Phelan, L. Landau and A. Olinsky (Blackwell, 1990)

8 Crying

Crying is the commonest way that an infant or young child communicates either need or distress. It is normal in the newborn and usually indicates hunger, thirst or need of a cuddle. Later it may be due to boredom, frustration, separation or pain. The amount of crying usually lessens by about three months, when the infant has learned that smiles get attention and that thumb-sucking soothes. By six months of age the infant has learned to use crying to attract attention. Some babies cry a lot more than others, possibly because they are oversensitive to stimuli of any sort, including their parents' response. As the crying continues, parental anxiety increases, the child then becomes worried and the crying can worsen. If this vicious circle continues, the child may be in danger of being physically abused.

There is a problem in defining what is excessive or frequent crying. Most people would agree that crying for more than three hours per day for more than three days per weeks for more than three weeks is outside the norm. Prolonged acute crying which does not respond to feeding and comforting is also abnormal. In most cases, the carer is able to identify the cause of crying, but the younger the child, the more difficult is the interpretation of the cry. There are two broad groups of crying behaviour which cause parents to look for help – persistent acute crying, and prolonged chronic crying (Fig. 8.1).

Persistent acute crying

History

Evaluation of the child presenting with acute persistent crying depends on the age of the child, and whether the child is well or ill (Table 8.1). The history will produce the most useful information.

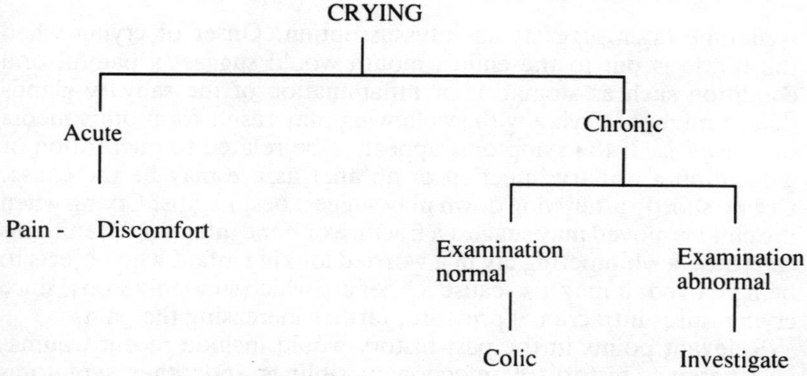

Fig. 8.1 Diagnostic pathway for crying

A better history will be obtained if it is elicited in a calm, unhurried, non-judgemental fashion. Appearing to be rushed or irritable is of no help to the parents, the distressed child or indeed the doctor. Observation of the parents and of the parent – child interaction during history taking is very important.

Table 8.1 Causes of acute crying

Central nervous system	Tumour, subdural haematoma.
Cardiovascular	Supraventricular tachycardia, heart failure.
ENT	Otitis media, laryngeal abrasion.
GIT	Stomatitis, oesophageal reflux, inguinal hernia, anal fissure, constipation, intussusception, lactose intolerance, cow's milk protein intolerance.
GUT	Obstruction (vesicoureteric, posterior urethral valve), urinary tract infection.
Musculoskeletal	Fracture, arthritis, haematoma.
Skin	Pruritic rash (eczema, scabies, etc.).
Others	Glaucoma, fetal alcohol syndrome, occult malignancy, drug withdrawal.

Most of these conditions can be diagnosed after a full physical examination and minimal laboratory or radiological tests.

The pattern of the crying can help indicate a diagnosis. Intermittent episodes of severe crying associated with sweating and pallor of sudden onset stopping in five to ten minutes only to be repeated sometime later suggests an intussusception. Onset of crying when the bottle is put to the child's mouth would suggest a painful oral condition such as stomatitis or inflammation of the salivary glands due to mumps. Crying with swallowing may result from otitis media or tonsillitis. If the symptoms appear to be related to micturition or defecation a urinary infection or an anal fissure may be the cause. Crying shortly after lying down may suggest oesphagitis. Crying when the child is moved may suggest a fracture or bone infection. Meningitis can cause a whimpering cry in a worried looking infant who objects to being moved; it may also cause a brief cry which suddenly stops, since crying raises intracranial pressure, further increasing the pain.

Relevant points in the past history would include recent trauma, vaccinations, history of infection in siblings and other symptoms associated with crying. The family history may be relevant, e.g. sickle cell disease. The child's bowel habit may give clues – diarrhoea may cause perianal soreness when associated with lactose intolerance and constipation may be associated with an anal fissure.

Examination

It is extremely important to gain the trust and co-operation of both the child and the parents. The child will be frightened not only by pain but by the unfamiliar surroundings, the doctor and the company of his parents whom he knows are anxious. Parents in turn will not trust the doctor if they sense hostility or lack of empathy. Some worried parents become aggressive. Five minutes spent calming parents and their crying child will make it much more likely that a satisfactory history and examination will be available. It is important to respect modesty in the older child. The scheme of examination should be very flexible and can be carried out with the child on the parents' lap or even standing. The order of examination will depend on the child's age, condition and site of pain. In the rare instance that the child is so distressed that examination is impossible, sedation with morphine or pethidine may be considered. Sedatives such as diazepam or trimeprazine may paradoxically worsen the child's agitation.

It is wise always to examine the non-painful areas first. Use of a spatula may not be necessary as the throat can often be adequately visualised when the child is crying. When examining the ears, most infants and children will stay still without restraint. If a rectal examination is carried out it should be done slowly, using the little finger. Throughout the examination it is helpful to talk to the child and to encourage the parents to distract him.

Abdominal palpation may be very difficult if the child is crying. It may still, however, be possible to elicit tenderness during inspiration. Sometimes, using the child's hand to palpate may be helpful. If the examination has been unsatisfactory examine the child again when he or she is asleep, having left the abdomen exposed. When the genitalia are being examined, inspection and very gentle, palpation should be all that is necessary. The vagina can be examined with the child on the couch or the parent's knee in either prone, supine or lateral position. Normal daylight gives better illumination than artificial light and the child's hands should be used to separate her labia. Rectal temperature is the quickest and most accurate way of recording body temperature.

Investigations

Where the cause of pain is not evident on clinical assessment further investigation is warranted. This will depend on the clinical presentation. Where infection is suspected a full blood count, urine and blood culture should be carried out. X-rays may be indicated if there is any suspicion of trauma. If intra-abdominal pathology is suspected, abdominal ultrasound is probably the quickest way of diagnosing intussusception. Barium or air enema can be used to treat. In the vast majority the clinical assessment coupled with these investigations will allow a diagnosis to be made. It is important to remember that the child must be given adequate analgesia whether or not a diagnosis has been made.

Prolonged chronic crying

The distinction between normal and abnormal crying behaviour depends on parents' perception and interpretation of their child's crying behaviour. Parents who look for help are usually correct in judging that their child cries a lot, though they may overestimate the length of time crying. There is no doubt that some infants cry longer, louder and more piercingly than others. Whether this is due to temperament, to efforts to communicate an unmet desire, or partly as a reaction to parental anxiety is unknown. Excessive crying may be more important for the distress and loss of self-confidence it causes parents than for its effect on the infant. Nevertheless, parental frustration may result in physical abuse of the child. An organic cause for crying is more likely if the crying is continuous rather than intermittent, if the child is inconsolable, or ill. A full clinical evaluation is important not only to exclude physical problems but also to relieve parents' fear of underlying serious illness.

Infantile colic is a behavioural syndrome characterised by excessive crying, which is paroxysmal in nature, more likely to occur in the evenings and without identifiable cause. It affects otherwise healthy infants between 2 weeks and 4 months. It is a diagnosis of exclusion. Colic affects some 10–15 per cent of all infants and it is equally common in breast and bottlefed infants. It usually begins in the first month of life. In individual babies it usually occurs at the same time each day, frequently in the afternoon or evening. The natural history is for gradual decline from about three months of age, though some infants may continue for up to a year. In some, crying episodes are associated with flexion of the legs, abdominal distension and the passage of excess wind. The infant may be very difficult to console during such an episode. By the time parents look for help they will usually have tried changing feeds and non-proprietary medications. Despite the ongoing symptoms these children usually thrive normally.

Though the cause of colic is not known there is no shortage of theories. These can be broken down into gastrointestinal and behavioural theories. Both seem to have an equal number of factors supporting and refuting their roles. Some workers believe that colic is a manifestation of food allergy and some studies have shown a response to exclusion diets in a minority. More recently, a prospective study from Finland has shown an association between parental experience of stress during pregnancy and after birth and colic in the baby. This would tend to support the view that colic is associated with, or caused by, parental maladaptation or psychological problems, with parental stress being transferred to the infant.

Clinical evaluation

Careful and detailed clinical appraisal is therapeutic. Document the age of onset, the pattern of crying and other problems such as vomiting, diarrhoea, pallor or cyanosis. Previous treatments should be ascertained. The degree of parental stress caused by the infant's crying should be assessed. The child should be carefully examined, paying particular attention to growth. In the child with intermittent symptoms it is unlikely that any abnormality will be detected. Nevertheless, care shown in a full examination will help allay parental anxiety.

Management

The family with a colicky infant presents a major challenge. The key issues include providing support through information and conversation as well as giving encouragement to the parents about coping mechanisms and nurturing skills so that family life may be eased a little. It is important to emphasise positive, 'good enough' parenting rather than perfect parenting. The number and variety of treatment options is an eloquent testimony to their lack of efficacy. In desperation, however, 'trying something' may give the parents some hope during what is otherwise a difficult time. Among the approaches suggested are behavioural responses – ensure that the infant is not hungry, wet, cold or lonely and if crying persists, to leave the infant to cry for a set period of time, gradually increased. Changing the feed to soya or 'hypoallergenic' milk may help (or coincide with a spontaneous improvement!). Treatment directed towards oesophageal reflux has also been recommended. Some parents find that the child will go asleep in the back of a moving car and a device is available in North America which mimicks this motion. For children with 'malignant' colic some authorities suggest sedation. Admission to hospital may have a role in defusing potentially dangerous situations. In infants with colic, spontaneous improvement is the rule. Until such time as this occurs adequate hospital and community based support is important.

Key points

- Persistent acute crying is usually caused by pain.
- A child who begins crying when handled is ill.
- Crying for more than 3 hours per day, for more than 3 days per week, for more than 3 weeks can be described as 'colic'.
- The aetiology of colic is unknown.
- Time is the most effective cure for colic.

Useful literature

- Psychosocial predisposing factors for infantile colic, P. Rautava, H. Helenius and L. Lehtonen (*British medical journal*, vol. 307, pp. 600–603, 1993)
- Infant colic, is it a gut issue?, Miller A., Barr, R.G. (*Ped. Clin. Nth. Amer.*, 1991 6, vol. 38, pp. 1407–23)

9 Dyspnoea

Dyspnoea simply means shortness of breath and it occurs when breathing becomes a conscious effort. It is commonly but not always associated with tachypnoea or rapid breathing. The spectrum of severity may vary from mild dyspnoea on exertion to severe distress at rest. In the latter situation it is important to make a rapid clinical assessment so that appropriate management can be expedited rapidly.

Clinical assessment

The sudden appearance of dyspnoea in a child is alarming for parents and delay in seeking medical attention is unusual. The differential diagnosis for sudden onset of dyspnoea is quite wide (Fig. 9.1) and a clinical approach to elucidating the cause of the problem is outlined in Table 9.1. When sudden onset of dyspnoea is due to an upper airway problem, it is usually predominantly inspiratory in character and associated with stridor. With viral croup there is usually

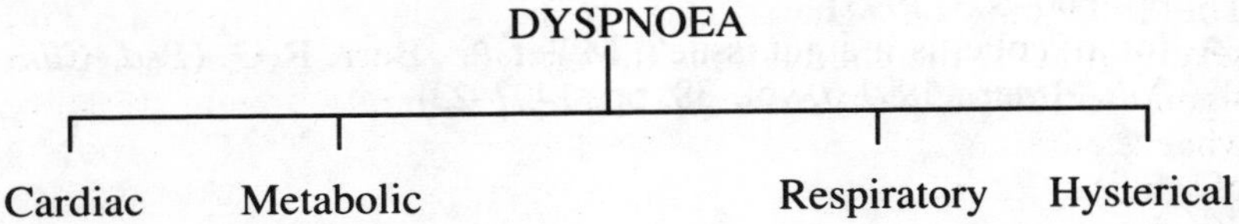

Fig. 9.1 Causes of acute dyspnoea

Table 9.1 Causes of acute dyspnoea

Upper airway	Croup Epiglottitis Foreign body
Lower respiratory tract	Asthma Pneumonia Bronchiolitis Pneumothorax Pleural effusion
Cardiac	Pericardial effusion Myocarditis Supraventricular tachycardia
Metabolic	Diabetic ketoacidosis Salicylate poisoning
Hysterical	

a history of coryzal symptoms for a few days prior to the onset of respiratory distress. The dyspnoea is associated with a barking cough and systemic upset is usually mild. It predominantly affects children in the preschool age group. Epiglottitis is a more serious condition but is much less common than viral croup. The causal agent is usually *Haemophilus influenzae* type B. It predominantly affects preschool children but may also occur in older children and adults. Onset is very rapid. The child appears pale, extremely ill and has a high fever. There is little or no cough but drooling is a prominent feature. Sudden onset of dyspnoea and stridor following a choking spell is strongly suggestive of a foreign body inhalation.

Dyspnoea due to acute pulmonary pathology such as asthma and bronchiolitis is predominantly expiratory in type. In acute asthma dyspnoea is usually accompanied by tachypnoea, tachycardia, signs of accessory muscle usage, intercostal and supraclavicular indrawing. The child may be agitated due to the anxiety or hypoxia. With severe attacks, the child adopts the upright posture and may have a significant pulsus paradoxus. Widespread inspiratory and expiratory wheezes are usually heard on auscultation of the chest. The nature of wheeze correlates poorly with the severity of the attack and in a life-threatening episode the chest may be silent.

Acute bronchiolitis most commonly occurs in infants under 6 months of age. The majority of cases are due to respiratory syncytial virus and epidemics occur during the winter months. Coryzal symptoms for a couple of days usually precede the development of an irritating cough, dyspnoea, tachypnoea and wheezing. The infant may have difficulty in feeding. They are usually not toxic, but the chest is hyperinflated and there is often retraction of the lower ribs during inspiration. Characteristically, widespread fine crackles are heard towards the end of inspiration and widespread wheezes occur on expiration. The liver may be pushed downwards because of the hyperinflated lungs and this may cause confusion with heart failure. The texture of the liver, however, is normal and there are no other signs of heart failure. In extreme cases respiratory failure may develop.

Dyspnoea with grunting respirations and flaring of the nostrils is common in childhood pneumonia. Other features of pneumonia are outlined in the chapter on cough. A large pneumothorax usually causes chest pain, cough and dyspnoea. The breath sounds are reduced on the side of the pleural air leak and there may be displacement of the trachea and apex beat to the opposite side. The most common cause is iatrogenic and it should be considered if a child suddenly deteriorates with increasing respiratory distress while receiving mechanical ventilation or after thoracocentesis. Dyspnoea may be due to the sudden appearance of a pleural effusion which may be associated with underlying cardiac or liver disorders or it may occur in association with pneumonia. The chest wall over a large effusion is dull to percussion and the breath sounds are diminished. The mediastinum may be pushed to the opposite side with large effusions. Dyspnoea due to pneumothorax or pleural effusion is classified with lower respiratory tract causes although it may not necessarily be predominantly expiratory in character.

Although any form of congenital heart disease with a large left to right shunt or conditions such as severe pulmonary valve stenosis will produce dyspnoea the symptom does not have an abrupt onset and will not be considered here.

The most common cause of a pericardial effusion in childhood is the postpericardiotomy syndrome. Effusions may be due to acute pericarditis or rheumatoid disease. With rapid accumulation of pericardial fluid the child develops acute dyspnoea. In chronic effusions, symptoms are vague and consist of lethargy, mild dyspnoea and abdominal swelling due to ascites. The pulse has a small volume and is reduced on inspiration. The jugular venous pulse is raised, the liver is enlarged and the heart sounds appear distant.

Children with acute myocarditis usually have a prodromal illness consisting of malaise and myalgia, possibly with some vomiting and diarrhoea. This is followed after a couple of days by dyspnoea or, in severe cases, sudden collapse with the development of cardiogenic shock. Examination reveals evidence of heart failure.

Table 9.2 Investigations of acute dyspnoea

Chest X-ray
Pulse
Arterial blood gas
Pulmonary function tests
ECG and rhythm strip
Laryngobronchoscopy under anaesthesia
Echocardiogram
Blood glucose
Salicylate level

Prolonged attacks of supraventricular tachycardia present with cough and dyspnoea due to the left heart failure and vomiting and abdominal pain due to hepatic engorgement. During an attack the patient is pale with a small volume and rapid regular pulse rate. Examination between attacks is normal unless there is underlying heart disease which is present in 20–30 per cent of patients.

Not all patients with sudden onset of dyspnoea have cardiac or respiratory problems. Deep sighing inspiration and expiration or Kussmaul breathing is associated with a low arterial PH. The respiratory amplitude is often markedly increased and is classically seen in diabetic ketoacidosis and salicylate poisoning. Hysterical dyspnoea is uncommon and is a diagnosis of exclusion. There must be no clinical evidence of an underlying organic disorder and the child may have other symptoms of anxiety. The respiratory pattern is often typical, consisting of deep breathing with a sudden holding of the breath after about every sixth breath. Occasionally hyperventilation may be severe enough to produce tetany.

Investigation

Unless the clinical assessment suggests that the dyspnoea is due to an upper airway problem, a chest X-ray is mandatory. If the child is acutely distressed pulse oximetry is a useful non-invasive method of monitoring oxygenation. Arterial blood gas sampling is a painful procedure and should not be performed lightly. Even in the severely dyspnoeic child with acute severe asthma, arterial blood gases at the time of presentation are not necessarily helpful in management. They frequently reveal quite marked hypoxia with or without carbon dioxide retention but the severity of the initial blood gas disturbance does not necessarily predict outcome and response to treatment. An arterial blood gas should certainly be performed if the child is not responding to standard treatment or if he or she is tiring and developing signs of respiratory failure.

Pulmonary function tests, particularly peak expiratory flow rates and forced expiratory volume in one second, are useful in the assessment of acute asthma but co-operation with these tests is impossible in a young child. Normal values for peak expiratory flow rates are available for children from two and a half years of age upwards although the majority of children under four will not perform the manoeuvre adequately during the acute attack. A standard ECG and rhythm strip should be done if the clinical assessment suggests a cardiac cause for the dyspnoea.

If epiglottitis or foreign body inhalation are suspected in a dyspnoeic child an urgent laryngobronchoscopy under anaesthesia should be performed by an experienced anaesthetist. An ENT surgeon should be on standby to perform an emergency tracheostomy if the child cannot be intubated. All invasive investigations should be withheld until the child has been examined under anaesthesia and the airway secured if necessary. The distress caused by a painful procedure such as the insertion of an intravenous line may precipitate complete airway obstruction in a child with epiglottitis.

Echocardiography is the most useful investigation if pericardial effusion or myocarditis are suspected. If there is no evidence of cardiac or pulmonary disease, blood gas should be performed and further investigations such as urea, electrolytes, blood sugar and salicylate levels will depend upon the clinical presentation.

Management

The management of a child who suddenly becomes dyspnoeic depends on the underlying cause of the problem but a number of general principles can be applied to any child who presents with this symptom. If the child is dyspnoeic at rest at he should be nursed in either an intensive care or high dependency area where constant monitoring and observation are available. As hypoxia frequently coincides with dyspnoea, humidified oxygen should be administered when the child presents, even before a specific diagnosis has been made. This measure often produces a significant clinical improvement and allows the doctor time to make a quick appraisal of the situation and instigate specific treatment. Some investigations are time consuming and their performance should not delay treatment although management may need to be adjusted depending on the results.

The management of the child with dyspnoea due to an upper airway problem is discussed in the chapter on stridor. Oxygen, regular nebulised bronchodilators and systemic corticosteroids are the mainstay of management of acute asthma. In severe cases intravenous aminophylline or intravenous salbutamol may be necessary, mechanical ventilation is rarely required.

The choice of antibiotic treatment in a child with pneumonia is guided by epidemiological considerations. Culture of the offending organism in blood is unlikely, and sputum is difficult to obtain in the young child. The possibility of chlamydia should be considered in a young infant with pneumonia and the treatment of choice is erythromycin. In the preschool age group *Haemophilus influenzae* or pneumococcus are likely and amoxycillin is the first line drug. A lobar pneumonia, particularly if associated with herpes labialis, is likely to be due to pneumococcus and penicillin is the drug of choice. *Mycoplasma pneumoniae* is the most frequent cause of pneumonia in children aged five to 15 years and erythromycin is the drug of choice.

Bronchiolitis is managed supportively – maintain oxygenation and hydration, treat secondary infection. Trials of bronchodilator therapy and systemic steroids have produced disappointing results in patients with acute viral bronchiolitis. A number of small clinical trials have been carried out using the antiviral drug ribavarin in nebulised form and results to date suggest that it is of some benefit. Treatment, however, is very expensive and most units restrict its use to patients with very severe bronchiolitis or bronchiolitis with underlying cardiorespiratory problems such as bronchopulmonary dysplasia or congenital heart disease. Conservative management is inappropriate in patients with dyspnoea due to pneumothorax, pleural or pericardial effusions and drainage is recommended in each case.

In acute myocarditis diuretics should be given, digoxin is used if there is ongoing impairment of left ventricular function. A dopamine infusion may be required if cardiogenic shock develops or there is a poor response to diuretic therapy. Supraventricular tachycardia can usually be terminated by various measures which induce vagal stimulation. In infancy immersion in iced water is most effective. Cardioversion is simple and effective, where the situation is critical. Intravenous adenosine is a safe and effective drug in terminating an episode but the relapse rate is high. Digoxin is still a valuable drug in the management of supraventricular tachycardia, particularly in infancy, and it is effective in suppressing further episodes.

The management of the child with dyspnoea due to acidosis is directed at the underlying cause. Hysterical dyspnoea can be difficult to treat and if an explanation for the problem and reassurance are not sufficient a psychological referral may be necessary.

Key points

- Quantify dyspnoea (e.g. dyspnoea talking versus dyspnoea running).
- If in doubt, give oxygen.
- Cyanosis is a late sign of hypoxia.
- Dyspnoea is not always respiratory.
- Oxygen is the most important drug in the management of bronchiolitis.

Useful literature

- *Respiratory illness in children*, 3rd edition, P. Phelan, L. Landau and A. Olinsky (Blackwell, 1990)
- Supraventricular tachycardia: diagnosis and current acute management, J. Till and E. Shinebourne (*Archives of diseases in childhood*, vol. 66, pp. 647–52, 1991)
- *Heart disease in paediatrics*, 3rd edition, S. Jordan and O. Scott (Butterworth, 1989)

10 Fever

Background

Fever is an elevation in body temperature due to a change in the heat regulatory set point in the hypothalamus. Normal body temperature is maintained within a 1.5 °C range of 37 °C. Temperatures in excess of 38.3 °C are generally abnormal. Temperature may be measured in the axilla of the mouth or the rectum. Rectal temperature is the most accurate. Axillary temperature may be up to 1 ° lower than core temperature and oral temperature may be lowered if the patient is tachypnoeic. Body temperature is maintained by balancing the heat generation, conservation and loss mechanisms. Heat is generated by increased cellular metabolism, muscle activity and involuntary shivering. Heat is conserved by peripheral vasoconstriction and heat preference behaviour. Heat loss is modulated through vasodilation, sweating and cold preference behaviour.

Fever is stimulated by an endogenous pyrogen. This causes hypothalamic mediated prostaglandin release, which upregulates the temperature set point. Infections are the commonest cause of fever but other influences such as tissue injury, malignancy, drugs, immunological and inflammatory diseases, endocrine and metabolic conditions can all result in fever. In rare instances, fever is factitious.

Fever as a response to infection occurs in all mammals, though the biological value of this is not clear. A fever, in itself, is associated with malaise and may trigger febrile convulsions. A very high temperature can interfere with other body systems.

The evaluation of fever in children invariably provokes a search for infectious disease. Whilst there are other causes, these are generally rare and usually present with prolonged fever of unknown origin. The major tasks in assessing an infant or child with fever is to decide whether the infection is local or systemic, trivial or serious.

Infants and children under 2 years of age present a particular problem. The risk of serious bacterial illness is greatest in early childhood. They are unlikely to have specific symptoms and clinical examination is often unhelpful.

Assessment of children under 2 years

This is the age group with the greatest mortality and morbidity from infectious disease. The higher the temperature and the younger the child, the more likely that there is serious illness. Because of the limited communication skills of this age group it is necessary to use 'veterinary' skills in assessment. The Babycheck is a recently devised scoring system to help with this particular problem, though it is not limited to the assessment of febrile infants. Acute illness observation scales (AIOS) are a further refinement of clinical assessment to help deal with this age group.

Try to obtain details of the onset of fever and whether there were concomitant symptoms. Babies with serious illness are usually reluctant to feed. Parents frequently notice that the child 'is not himself' and lacks interest in his surroundings. The combination of a child who is drowsy but irritable when handled is particularly suggestive of meningitis. Try to record the amount of feed taken in the previous day and also any change in the pattern of stool or micturition. Vomiting may accompany gastroenteritis, urinary infection or indeed meningitis. A change in the baby's cry may indicate pain.

Enquire as to the presence of illness in the home or recent contact with infectious disease. Record the child's immunisation status and the timing of the last vaccine. Recent antibiotic treatment can make clinical assessment more difficult since it may mask symptoms.

Whilst taking the history observe the child in the mother's arms. Seriously ill infants do not smile and show little or no interest in their surroundings, or in strangers. They tend to be hypotonic and in severe cases may be totally oblivious to their surroundings. Record the temperature, pulse and respiratory rate. The presence of nasal flaring, moderate or severe chest recession would indicate respiratory illness. If the hands and feet are cool and cyanosed with diminished capillary refill time this may indicate dehydration or peripheral shut-down associated with central pyrexia. Look for any signs of a rash, particularly petechial or Koplik spots. A bulging fontanelle, opisthotonic posturing and obvious neck stiffness are absent in the early stages of meningitis and their presence usually indicates advanced pathology with a poor prognosis despite treatment. The infant with mastoiditis will have asymmetric 'bat' ear. Where there is osteomyelitis or septic arthritis there will be pseudoparesis and exquisite local tenderness. Serious infection in the blood, urine, lungs, and spinal fluid may not be associated with specific signs or symptoms unless very advanced.

The acute illness observation scales (AIOS) were developed by McCarthy *et al.* in the 1980s and are a useful guide to the assessment of small children with fever (Table 10.1). Scores are allocated for each item. A total score over ten is predictive of serious illness. Unfortunately, there is no substitute for experience in evaluating this age group. If the clinician is relatively new to paediatrics he should pay great attention to mother's intuition and particularly to the impression of experienced paediatric nurses. In general, particularly in the very young infants, it is best to err on the side of caution with a low threshold for investigation and treatment.

Investigation

The necessity for and the extent of investigation will depend upon the clinican's decision as to whether there is a clear explanation for the fever or if it is felt likely that there is serious bacterial infection present. If the baby is clearly very ill then full 'septic screen' is appropriate. In cases where the presentation is not so clearcut, investigations may help the clinician decide whether further tests or treatment are necessary. A full blood count and blood film will be the single most helpful test in this regard.

Serious bacterial sepsis is often associated with a very low or a very high white cell count, dominant neutrophilia and elevated numbers of immature neutrophils. A white cell count less than 5000 or greater than 15 000, with more than 1500 'band' forms suggests sepsis. The platelet count may be diminished where there is disseminated intravascular coagulopathy; elevated platelet count may be associated with inflammation or recent bleeding. Anaemia would usually indicate a longstanding problem. Measurements of erythrocyte sedimentation rate (ESR) and C-reactive protein (CRP) are helpful in some situations but in general rarely help the clinician with a diagnostic dilemma. Urine that is 'crystal clear' is almost certainly not infected. Cloudiness in the urine may be due to infection or more commonly to urate crystals. Urine microscopy showing heavy pyuria suggests infection. The blood sugar may be significantly elevated in the child with serious illness as part of the 'stress' response.

When the clinician is confident that there is serious illness present, blood cultures should be drawn, urine sent for microscopy and a chest X-ray requested. The indications for lumbar puncture remain

Table 10.1 Observation scales for febrile children (McCarthy *et al.*, 1982)

Observation Item	1 Normal	3 Moderate impairment	5 Severe impairment
Quality of cry	Strong, normal, or content and not crying	Whimpering or sobbing	Weak or moaning or highpitched
Reaction to parent stimulation	Cries briefly then stops. Content and not crying	Cries off and on	Continual cry or hardly responds
State variation	If awake – stays awake. If asleep and stimulated, wakes up quickly	Eyes close briefly awake or awakes with prolonged stimulation	Falls asleep or will not rouse
Colour	Pink	Pale extremities or acrocyanosis. Mottled or ashen	Pale or cyanotic
Hydration	Skin normal, eyes normal and mucous membranes moist	Skin, eyes normal and mouth slightly dry	Skin doughy or tented, dry mucous membranes and/or sunken eyes
Response (talk, smile) to social approach	Smiles or alerts (< 2 mo)	Brief smile or alerts briefly (< 2 mo); expressionless or no alerting (< mo)	No smile Face anxious

somewhat controversial. Some authors advocate lumbar punctures in all infants under a year with significant pyrexia, others reserving this investigation for specific instances. In experienced hands, lumbar puncture is a safe procedure and is not especially traumatic in infants. A low threshold for the performance of lumbar puncture is appropriate. 'If the diagnosis of meningitis crosses your mind, do an LP.' Infants with meningitis are usually quite toxic and apathetic and the procedure is rarely difficult but conversely the child without meningitis is likely to be vigorous and to present a 'moving target'. Chest X-ray is necessary since clinical signs of pneumonia may be entirely absent despite extensive consolidation radiographically.

Management

Local cause Where a child has an obvious focus for infection, e.g. otitis media, tonsillitis, urinary infection, then appropriate antibiotics should be administered and modified in the light of culture results.

Serious infection with no obvious focus

Cultures should be drawn and the patient treated empirically with broad spectrum antibiotics. The combination of ampicillin and gentamicin is often used in hospitalised infants; more recently third generation cephalosporins such as ceftriaxone have been used for both inpatients and outpatients with unexplained high fever.

Serious infection with a known cause

The management of meningitis, osteomyelitis and pneumonia should be dictated by local protocols.

Management of fever

A febrile infant should be given a liberal fluid intake and excess bedding and clothing removed. Where an electric fan is used it is important that this is not directed at the infant, since this can cause peripheral vasoconstriction and paradoxically raise the temperature. Similarly, with tepid sponging, attention to detail is important. If the water used for sponging is too cold vasoconstriction may result. The aim of tepid sponging is to increase blood flow to the periphery, thereby facilitating cooling. Paracetamol or ibuprofen may be given to cause a reduction in temperature. It is thought that these act by inhibiting prostaglandin which mediates the change at the heat regulatory set point. Aspirin is no longer used in children under 12 years because of the risk of causing Reye's syndrome.

Assessment of children over 2 years

In this age group children are more likely to have localising symptoms, e.g. dysuria, pleuritic pain, headache. Enquire as to the onset and duration of the fever and the presence of associated symptoms. Immunisation status, exposure to infectious disease, and recent antibiotic treatment are all relevant. The number and age of siblings and whether the child attends school, creche or playgroup may give a clue as to the source of infection. Family history is relevant where immunodeficiency is suspected.

Clinical examination should be comprehensive, paying particular attention to likely foci of infection. Examine the ear drums and the throat and look for herpes labialis which is sometimes a clue to pneumonia. Is there any rash? Children with lobar pneumonia may have little by way of clinical signs but usually complain of pleuritic pain, have a shallow cough and nasal flaring. Factitious fever does not cause an elevated pulse rate.

Investigations

Since the risk of fulminating sepsis is less in older children, one could be somewhat more circumspect about the choice of investigations and the need for 'blind' antibiotic treatment. Management of fever itself follows similar lines to those outlined for infants.

Key points

- The higher the fever and the younger the infant – the greater the risk of serious infection.
- Food and play are top of the child's agenda – disinterest in one or both is significant.
- A smile excludes meningitis in infancy.
- If a baby looks worried - this is not neuroticism!
- In factitious fever the pulse is not elevated.

Useful literature

- Outpatient management without antibiotics of fever in selected

infants, M. Baker, L. Bell and J. Avner (*New England journal of medicine*, vol. 329, pp. 1437–41, 1993)
- Babycheck, a scoring system to grade the severity of acute systemic illness in babies under six months old, C. Marley *et al.* (*Archives of disease in childhood*, vol. 66, 100–5, 1991)
- Observations scales to identify serious illness in febrile children, P. McCarthy *et al.* (*Paediatrics*, vol. 70, 802–9, 1982)

11 Haematuria

Introduction

Haematuria is one of those symptoms or signs which usually result in children being brought to the doctor promptly. Increasingly widespread usage of dipstick tests results in the documentation of microscopic haematuria. Bleeding from the urinary tract is a cause of understandable concern to parents and therefore requires an explanation.

Clearly it is important for clinicians to separate haematuria into causes which are clinically common and relevant, but also to be aware of rarer serious causes. Minimal investigation will be required in most cases but occasionally a renal biopsy is necessary . The term idiopathic haematuria should rarely, if ever, be used.

History

The history will need to focus on the presenting symptom and questions are formulated to take account of likely diagnoses. First exclude spurious haematuria. Florid discoloration of urine can be due to ingestion of beetroot, drugs such as rifampicin, the presence of urates, haemoglobin or myoglobin in the urine. Ask for the colour of the urine, whether it is red, smoky or black. If there is pain try to localise this. Define whether the haematuria is persistent or intermittent whether there is any bleeding elsewhere or associated rash or joint pains. The relationship to exercise or recent tonsillitis is relevant. A family history of haematuria, deafness, renal failure, sickle cell disease or autoimmune disease is important. Recent foreign travel may indicate a tropical infection. Recent haemorrhagic diarrhoea may herald haemolytic uraemic syndrome.

Physical examination

Examine for the presence of oedema or hypertension. Suprapubic or loin tenderness will indicate urinary infection or occasionally calculus. The presence of a purpuric rash may suggest systemic vasculitis (Henoch–Schonlein purpura). A general examination may indicate anaemia suggesting a haemoglobinopathy or other chronic disorder.

Examination of the urine can be considered under the physical examination as it is a fundamental and very helpful way of categorising haematuria. Examination for the presence of red cells will confirm whether there is indeed a problem. Where casts are seen this clearly indicates a glomerular lesion and an accordingly different set of priorities for investigation (Fig. 11.1).

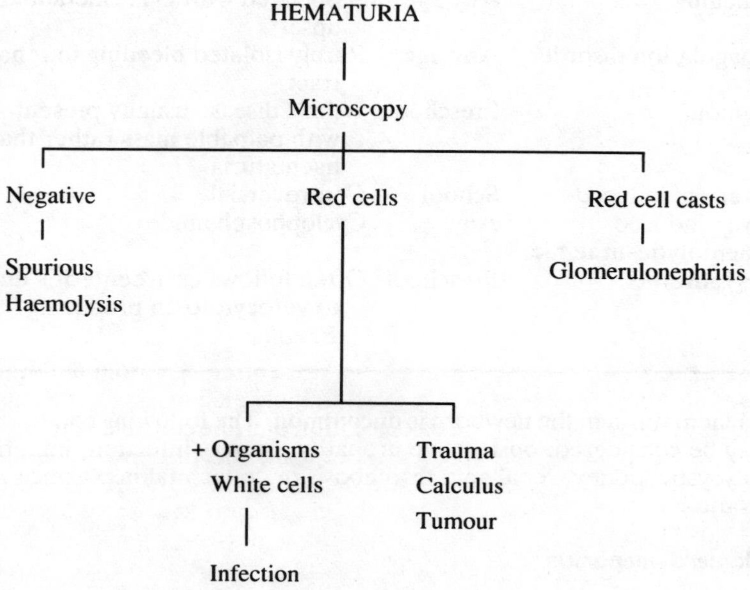

Fig. 11.1 Diagnostic pathway for haematuria

Clinical interpretation

The basic rules in haematuria are that common things are considered first, that deductive logic be applied to the findings on history, examination and urine microscopy and that either a clinical diagnosis is reached or a couple of likely possibilities are entertained. Blanket investigation protocols are unpleasant for children, expensive and represent poor clinical judgement. The most common explanations of acute haematuria are urinary tract infection, glomerulonephritis and trauma. Possible causes, ages and associated factors are shown in Table 11.1.

Table 11.1 Causes of haematuria

Causes	*Age*	*Comment*
Urinary tract infection	Any	Commonest, upper or lower tract
Trauma	School	Must be fairly severe to induce bleeding
Glomerulonephritis	School	Acute or chronic; several types
Calculus	Any age	Associated with UTI, metabolic upset
Coagulation disorder	Any age	Rarely isolated bleeding in renal tract
Tumour	Preschool	Wilm's disease usually present with palpable mass rather than haematuria
Exercise induced	School	Controversial
Drug induced	Any	Cyclophosphamide
Haemolytic–uraemic syndrome	Preschool	Often follows gastroenteritis due to verocytotoxin producing *E. coli*.

Haematuria in the newborn is uncommon. The following conditions may be considered: obstructive uropathy, urinary infection, infantile polycystic kidney, renal vein thrombosis or congenital nephrotic syndrome.

Glomerulonephritis

The presence of haematuria with casts and proteinuria could be called 'nephritic urine'. This could be due to acute poststreptococcal glomerulonephritis, Henoch–Schonlein nephritis, IgA nephropathy, hereditary nephritis (Alport syndrome), systemic lupus erythematosus, or rarer types of nephritis.

Investigation

The extent of the investigation will depend on the likely diagnosis. Confirmation of a urinary infection will prompt imaging of upper (ultrasound and plain abdominal radiograph) and sometimes lower urinary tract, with follow-up to ensure clearance of infection. A finding of glomerulonephritis will lead to measurement of serial renal function and quantitative estimation of proteinuria. Serum creatinine is a simple and reliable measure. Estimation of ESR, antistreptolysin titre and complement level will give further useful information.

Renal calculi are uncommon in children in the developed world but are seen where there is obstruction or chronic infection. Idiopathic hypercalcuria is being increasingly recognised in children. Further detailed investigation is appropriate but is beyond the remit of this chapter.

The place of renal biopsy remains problematic, but it is reasonable to consider biopsy if there is a nephritic or nephrotic picture with no clinical diagnosis, where haematuria exists despite extensive investigation, if there is a family history of renal failure, deafness or recurrent haematuria or there is persistent haematuria for 6–12 months.

Key points

- Other causes of red or dark urine must be considered.
- Tiny amounts of blood (0.25 ml in 250 ml urine) can darken the urine.
- A dipstick test positive for blood is not diagnostic of a UTI.
- The combination of haematuria + proteinuria + casts points to a glomerular lesion.
- Haematuria *per se* rarely if ever results in anaemia in childhood.
- Wilm's tumour rarely presents as haematuria.
- It takes severe renal trauma to produce haematuria from a normal kidney.
- Conversely haematuria following minor or mild trauma may suggest a renal cyst or pelviureteric junction obstruction.
- Acute glomerulonephritis does not usually require a renal biopsy, unless clinically severe; chronic glomerulonephritis may require biopsy, if only for diagnostic and prognostic purposes.

Useful literature

- Haematuria, S. Meadow. In: *Clinical paediatric nephrology*, R. Postlethwaite (ed.) (Wright, 1986)
- *A handbook of renal investigations in children*, C. Taylor and S. Chapman (Wright, 1989)
- The investigation of haematuria in children, R. White (*Archives of diseases in childhood*, vol. 64, pp. 159–165, 1989)
- An office approach to haematuria and proteinuria, M. Norman (*Paediatric clinics of North America*, vol. 34, pp. 545–60, 1987)

12 Jaundice

Jaundice may be due to accumulation of either conjugated or unconjugated bilirubin (Table 12.1). Hepatitis A is the major cause of jaundice in older children. However, jaundice may be the earliest or only sign of chronic liver disease and therefore requires careful evaluation.

Assessment of the jaundiced child

History

Evaluation of the child with jaundice begins with an accurate history. It is important to document the time of onset and course of jaundice. Nausea, vomiting, anorexia and abdominal pain may precede jaundice in infectious hepatitis. Sudden onset of jaundice suggests a viral or drug aetiology. Persistent mild jaundice of varying intensity suggests haemolysis or Gilbert's disease. The presence of dark urine and pale stools may precede hepatocellular or obstructive jaundice by several days. In haemolytic jaundice the stools are well pigmented.

Non-specific symptoms such as anorexia, abdominal pain, pruritus, bleeding or abdominal distension may indicate the presence of chronic liver disease. It is important to document any contact with infectious diseases, exposure to drugs, toxins, parenteral infusions or recent general anaesthetic. A family history of consanguinity, unexplained liver or neurological disease, haemolytic disorders, autoimmune disease or Wilson's disease should be noted.

Clinical evaluation

General examination The nutritional state of the child will often indicate the severity of underlying liver disease. Failure to thrive may be secondary to chronic liver disease and associated fat malabsorption due to inadequate bile secretion. The weight and height at presentation should be compared to previous measurements. Subcutaneous fat can be assessed clinically in the thigh, gluteal, biceps and triceps areas. It can also be measured using skin calipers. Percentile charts for skinfold thickness are available.

Anaemia may be seen in association with haemolysis or cirrhosis. The presence of limb oedema probably indicates hypoalbuminaemia

Table 12.1 Causes of jaundice in children over the age of 1 year

Unconjugated
Haemolysis, e.g. sickle cell disease
Gilbert's
Crigler–Najjar
Conjugated
Infection
Hepatitis A,B,C,D,E
Epstein–Barr virus
Cytomegalovirus
Varicella
Bacterial infection
Tuberculosis
Metabolic
1-antitrypsin
Wilson's disease
Cystic fibrosis
Glycogen storage disease type IV
Miscellaneous
Dubin–Johnson syndrome
Rotor syndrome
Autoimmune hepatitis
Congenital hepatic fibrosis
Chronic obstruction
Drugs

which is usually a reflection of chronic, severe liver disease. Arthropathy may be a feature of autoimmune chronic active hepatitis or of hepatitis B infection.

Skin

Scratch marks, from intense itching due to bile salt retention, are often a feature of chronic liver disease. Spider naevi seen in chronic disease are reflections of altered oestrogen metabolism. They consist of a vascular malformation with a central venule supplying a number of radiating vessels. They are distributed within an area supplied by the superior vena cava. Bruising may indicate a clotting defect indicative of poor hepatic synthetic function, or be related to thrombocytopenia which occurs in association with hypersplenism. Xanthomas may be present and are due to increased serum cholesterol levels.

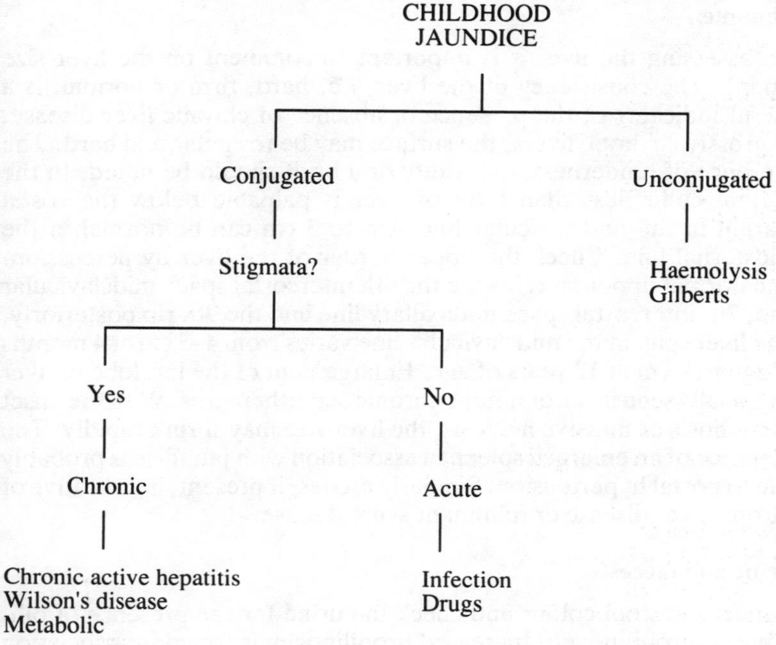

Fig. 12.1 Diagnostic pathway for jaundice beyond infancy

Hands

Clubbing of the fingers and toes may be a feature of any chronic liver disease. Palmar erythema is rare in children but when present, is most obvious over the thenar and hypothenar eminence and tips of fingers. Flapping tremor (asterixis) is rare in children and where present, indicates that the onset of encephalopathy is imminent.

Eyes

A careful eye examination can provide useful information especially if Kayser–Fleischer (KF) rings or cataracts are identified. Slit lamp examination is essential to document early KF rings. Although typically found in Wilson's disease, they can occur with prolonged cholestasis of any cause. Rarely, xanthomas of the eyelids may be found indicating hypercholesterolaemia.

Abdomen

On assessing the liver it is important to comment on the liver size (span). The consistency of the liver, i.e. hard, firm or normal, is a useful indicator of the presence or absence of chronic liver disease. In grossly cirrhotic livers, the surface may be irregular and hard. The presence of tenderness, pulsatility or a bruit should be noted. In the normal child, less than 1 cm of liver is palpable below the costal margin in the midclavicular line. Up to 3 cm can be normal in the midsternal line. Check the upper border of the liver by percussion. The normal upper margins are the 5th intercostal space midclavicular line, 7th intercostal space midaxillary line and the 9th rib posteriorly. The liver span in the midclavicular line varies from 4–5 cm at 4 months of age to 9 cm at 12 years of age. Enlargement of the left lobe of liver is typically seen in autoimmune chronic active hepatitis. With the onset of cirrhosis or massive necrosis, the liver size may shrink rapidly. The presence of an enlarged spleen in association with jaundice is probably due to portal hypertension. Similarly ascites, if present, is indicative of chronic liver disease or fulminant acute disease.

Urine and faeces

Inspect the stool colour and check the urine for the presence of bilirubin or urobilinogen. Increased urobilinogen is found in association with haemolysis. Persistent absence of urobilinogen is suggestive of biliary obstruction. Viral and drug associated hepatitis are characterised by early bilirubinuria.

Investigations (Table 12.2)

A full blood count, reticulocyte count and serum bilirubin with fractions (conjugated and unconjugated) are initially measured. Aminotransferases are intracellular enzymes found in most tissues (see 'Neonatal Cholestasis'). Increased aspartatate aminotransferase (AST) and alanine aminotransferase (ALT) therefore reflect hepatocellular damage. Transaminase levels are useful in following the

Table 12.2 Investigation of liver disease in children over 1 year of age

Haematology	*Renal*
FBC	Urea, creatinine
Coag. screen	Calcium, phosphate
Reticulocyte count	Blood gas
Coomb's test	
Liver profile	*Miscellaneous*
AST, ALT, Alk phos, GGT	Immunoglobulins
Albumin	Complement 3 & 4
Cholesterol, triglycerides	Tissue autoantibodies
Uric acid	Alpha fetoprotein
Magnesium	Alpha 1-antitrypsin – level/phenotype
Copper studies	Amino acids
Plasma copper	Lactate/pyruvate
Ceruloplasmin	Monospot test
24 hour urine pre & post penicillamine	Urine – organic acids
	Sweat test
	Vitamen levels
Virology	(if chronic liver disease)
Hepatitis A, B, C	A,D,E
Antibodies to HIV,	
CMV, EB	
Toxo, herpes, syphilis	
Radiological studies	
Abdominal US	
ERCP	
HIDA scan	

course of acute liver disease. Normal transaminases do not necessarily imply normal liver function. They are also of limited value in monitoring the progress of disease to cirrhosis.

Alkaline phosphatase isoenzymes are also widely distributed. Total levels are raised in childhood because of on-going bone growth. Levels increase when hepatic excretion is obstructed. Gamma glutamyl transpeptidase (GGT) is found throughout the biliary tree but is also present in many other organs. Therefore while serum GGT is useful in identifying children with biliary disease, it is very non-specific.

Serum albumin, together with the prothrombin time are indicators of the synthetic function of the liver and are therefore valuable tests for following severe liver disease. Abnormalities in serum cholesterol, triglycerides, calcium, phosphate, urea and creatinine may document secondary complications of liver disease.

Infections hepatitis

The hepatitis viruses A, B and C may cause a wide spectrum of liver disease ranging from asymptomatic mild inflammation to fulminant liver failure. Chronic infection occurs in some cases and may be subclinical or may progress to severe chronic liver disease.

Hepatitis A Measurement of hepatitis A specific IgM is the method of choice for the diagnosis of hepatitis A. IgG antibody persists indefinitely and is thought to be responsible for immunity following most infections. Hepatitis A never causes chronic liver disease.

Hepatitis B The serological response to hepatitis B virus infection (HBV) varies from patient to patient. Commonly there is a 'window' period between the disappearance of viral antigens and the appearance of antibodies. Some chronic carriers never mount an antibody response.

The first measurable antigens to appear in acute HBV infection are the Dane particle, HBV DNA polymerase and hepatitis B surface antigen (HBsAg). The appearance of these antigens may precede the development of symptoms or elevated levels of ALT. Hepatitis Be antigen (HBeAg) is usually detectable within a few weeks and correlates with high infectivity.

Approximately 4 weeks after the first detection of antigen, an antibody response begins with the appearance of IgM HBc (core) antibody. HBe antibody will later be detectable. Following recovery and clearance of the virus, serum will contain HBsAb which confers protection from reinfection. Some patients will fail to clear the virus and will remain infective. High infectivity is suggested by the coexistence of high titres of HBsAg, HBeAg and DNA polymerase – all of which imply continuing viral replication. Low titres of HBsAg together with HBe antibody indicate low infectivity and may be due to the incorporation of the viral DNA, which encodes for surface antigen, into the host genome.

Hepatitis D Delta hepatitis occurs only in association with hepatitis B and may be responsible for acute hepatitis or severe chronic liver disease in these patients. It is diagnosed by measuring delta antibody levels.

Hepatitis C Hepatitis C (HCV) is responsible for the majority of post-transfusion hepatitis, and a large proportion of sporadic 'non-A, non-B' hepatitis. It is possible to detect specific serum anti-HC antibodies based on recombinant proteins. Hepatitis C can also be diagnosed using PCR to detect HCV RNA sequences. Antibodies may not appear for several months after infection and false positive results may occur in patients with autoimmune chronic active hepatitis.

Leptospirosis may be associated with jaundice, but other features such as meningism and renal abnormalities are usually more prominent. Hepatitis may occur as part of infections mononucleosis (Epstein–Barr virus infection).

Wilson's disease

The diagnosis of Wilson's disease must be considered in any child over the age of five years with liver disease. It can mimic any form of parenchymal hepatic disorder from mild acute hepatitis to fulminant hepatic failure and cirrhosis. Whilst early diagnosis is imperative to prevent further cell damage, it is often difficult to make a definite diagnosis.

Caeruloplasmin is an alpha 2 globulin produced by the liver and acts as a carrier for copper. In Wilson's disease there is a deficiency of this protein. Low levels may also be seen, however, in heterozygotes and in conditions where protein is deficient, e.g. malnutrition, protein loosing enteropathy, nephrotic syndrome and hepatic insufficiency. The usefulness of caeruloplasmin levels is limited by the fact that it is an acute phase reactant and in 5–25 per cent of cases of Wilson's disease levels can be within the normal range. Similarly, serum copper estimation is of limited value in the diagnosis of Wilson's disease, as levels may be high, low or normal. In normal individuals urinary copper values are less than 0.6 μmol/24 hours. In Wilson's disease, more than 1.25 μmol per day of copper is excreted with values of up to 12.5 μmol per day being frequently found. However, urinary copper concentrations may also be increased in other chronic liver conditions, e.g. chronic active hepatitis. A 24 hour urinary copper excretion after a penicillamine challenge ($>$ 25 μmol/24 hours) is probably the best biochemical test to distinguish Wilson's disease from other chronic liver diseases.

Autoimmune chronic active hepatitis

Immunoglobulins The diagnosis of autoimmune chronic active hepatitis (ACAH) is suggested by a high concentration of immunoglobulin especially IgG, with levels in excess of 16 g/l. Elevated levels of IgG may also be found in sclerosing cholangitis.
Auto-antibodies A diagnosis of ACAH is further supported by the presence of non-organ specific autoantibodies (antinuclear factor, anti smooth muscle antibody, antimitochondrial antibody, liver-kidney microsomal antibodies (LKMA)) in the serum. Antinuclear factor and smooth muscle antibodies are also found in sclerosing cholangitis.

High titres of anti liver specific lipoprotein (LSP) antibody may be found in ACAH with levels decreasing in response to treatment. A close relationship has been demonstrated between serum concentrations of anti-LSP and the extent of periportal inflammation and necrosis on liver biopsy. Anti-LSP can appear transiently in hepatitis A and B infections.

Complement Seventy per cent of children with ACAH will have decreased levels of C4 with 20 per cent having low C3 levels. The underlying mechanism is unclear. Secondary impairment of hepatic synthesis or increased complement consumption by antibody-antigen reactions have been suggested.

Metabolic

Alpha 1-antitrypsin (A1AT) deficiency may present with chronic liver disease in childhood and adolescence. Children with evidence of chronic liver disease should have A1AT levels and phenotyping done (see 'Neonatal Hepatitis'). Cystic fibrosis should be considered in children with unexplained chronic liver disease.

Radiological evaluation

Ultrasound of liver and spleen

Ultrasound of liver, spleen and abdominal cavity is of limited value in diffuse liver disease. Increased echogenicity is found in association with a fatty liver. Dilated ducts may indicate obstruction. A choledochal cyst, calculi or sludge within the gallbladder may be identified. In patients with portal hypertension, ultrasound with Doppler is useful in assessing patency of the portal vein. It can also be used to evaluate the presence of collateral circulation.

Endoscopic retrograde cholangiopancreatography (ERCP)

ERCP allows visualisation of the intrahepatic and extrahepatic biliary tree. Radio-opaque dye is injected directly following cannulation of the ampulla of Vater using fibreoptic endoscopy. It is of value in patients with suspected sclerosing cholangitis, demonstrating areas of narrowing and dilatation of intrahepatic and extrahepatic bile ducts.

Liver biopsy

A liver biopsy should be considered in any patient with acute hepatitis which does not resolve within four weeks and is not attributable to infectious hepatitis. Biopsy at an earlier stage is indicated in the presence of chronic stigmata of liver disease, non-organ specific autoantibodies or high IgG concentration.

Management

As in cholestasis in infancy, attention should be focused on the general aspects of management of the older child paying particular attention to nutritional needs, vitamin deficiencies and symptoms of cholestasis (see Chap. 32). Children with fulminant hepatic failure require specialist assessment. Correction and prevention of hypoglycaemia, and electrolyte disturbances are essential prior to transfer to a specialist centre.

Children with hepatitis A should be treated symptomatically. At present children with hepatitis B are not given specific treatment although the use of interferon may be considered in specialised centres. There is as yet no specific treatment for hepatitis C.

The mainstay of treatment for auto-immune chronic active hepatitis (ACAH) is prednisolone. If steroid withdrawal is associated with a rise in serum transaminases, azothioprine is commenced. Regular full blood counts must be monitored to detect bone marrow suppression.

Wilson's disease is treated using D-penicillamine. It will stop progression of disease activity in patients with established liver disease. In patients unable to tolerate penicillamine, triethylene tetramine, a chelating agent, or zinc which antagonises copper absorption, can be used.

Patients with alpha 1-antitrypsin deficiency are treated symptomatically. Some of these children will ultimately require liver transplantation.

Liver transplantation

In spite of medical management certain children will develop progressive liver disease. It is important to identify those children in whom liver transplantation may be necessary. The 1 year survival rate for children following liver transplantation is now in excess of 85 per cent. A critical factor in liver transplantation is deciding the correct time to carry out the transplant procedure bearing in mind that many children with chronic liver disease will remain stable for months or years.

Key points

- Prothrombin time is the best indicator of progress in acute hepatic disease.
- Monitor and correct the potassium and sugar level in hepatic failure.
- Urinary copper excretion after penicillamine is the best test for Wilson's disease.
- Clinical stigmata, and hypoalbuminaemia imply that liver disease is chronic.
- Examination of the liver should document consistency as well as size.

Useful literature

- *Paediatric hepatology*, M. Tanner (Churchill Livingstone, 1989).
- *Paediatric gastrointestinal disease*, W. Walker, P. Durie, J. Hamilton, J. Walker Smith and J. Watkins (B.C. Decker, 1991)
- *Liver disorders in childhood*, A. Mowat (Butterworth, 1994)

13 Limp

The main diagnostic challenge of limp is in toddlers. Older children may not complain of limp as such – they will have a limp as a consequence of pain which they will readily describe. Consequently history and examination sequence will be quite different in preschool and schoolgoing children.

Limping toddlers

History

Define the onset of the symptom, whether it is worsening or improving. Establish clearly whether there was a preceding causative fall. Many toddlers suffer frequent minor falls and parents may mistakenly attribute the child's limp to a trivial fall and this can in turn lead the doctor to a false differential diagnosis. A fall can only be accepted as a cause of limp if one establishes clearly that the child was normally mobile, had a witnessed fall and since the fall has been limping. If such a historical sequence is established then one's clinical and radiological search is for a fracture. If not, the differential diagnosis is much broader. The diagnostic categories where there is no clear history of trauma would include:

1. Infection of bone or joint (septic arthritis or osteomyelitis). Enquire as to the child's temperature and general well-being. Is there pain in the absence of weight-bearing or pain during sleep?
2. Hip joint problems are common and these would include 'irritable hip'. This is also sometimes referred to as a transient synovitis. This would be the commonest cause of limp in toddlers. Perthe's

disease, which is due to aseptic necrosis of the femoral head, usually presents with a chronic history and is a common cause of limp. Late presenting congenital dislocation of the hip is rare.

3. Miscellaneous and unusual causes would include embedded foreign body, verruca, tumour of bone, painful groin due to problems other than the hip, e.g. incarcerated hernia or torsion of testis. Bone dysplasia such as osteoid osteoma or bony exostosis may also present with limp.

The age at which the child began to walk and whether the gait had been normal up to the onset of symptoms are clearly important. For instance, a limp beginning as the child begins to walk would strongly suggest a late presenting hip dysplasia. The family history is important since both hip dysplasia and Perthe's disease may be familial.

Examination

Try to get the child to walk if possible. Inspect the gait; how severe is the limp? Is the limp plantigrade? Does the child walk tip-toe or

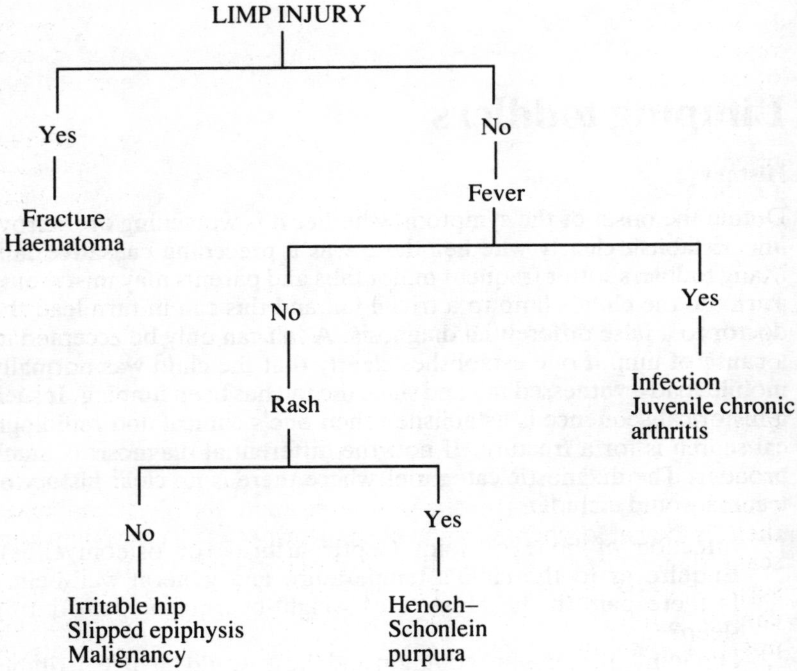

Fig. 13.1 Diagnostic pathway for limping child

on the heel of the limping leg? Children with painful hips limp tip-toe, holding the hip flexed and externally rotated. Walking on the heel suggests a painful sole or forefoot – inspect both lower limbs and compare. Swelling of the knee or ankle joints is usually obvious on inspection, unlike the hip joint, which is deeply situated. Inspect the child's posture – is the limping limb held in a particular position? The child who lies with hip and knee flexed and the hip externally rotated is localising his or her limp to hip pain. Expose the child from waist to foot. Limping toddlers are best examined on a parent's knee where they are reassured and most likely to be quiet.

Palpate both lower limbs lightly at first looking for areas of localised heat and tenderness. Next examine the hips. Always test the hip on the non-limping side first and then on the symptomatic side. With the knee flexed to 90° internally rotate the hip joint until the pelvis starts to tilt. If the hip joint is painful there will be painful limitation of internal rotation. Note the extent of limitation. Where sepsis is present there is usually gross limitation.

Investigation

If there is a positive localising sign, i.e. bony tenderness, X-ray the relevant area. Always X-ray in two planes at right angles to each other. X-rays of the hips should include both hips and a lateral film of the symptomatic hip.

Fractures are not always obvious in toddlers. Subperiosteal crack fractures, usually of the tibia, are common and may not be evident radiologically until a week to 10 days after the fracture, when subperiosteal calcification becomes evident. Accordingly, if the history is strongly suggestive of fracture, it is worthwhile repeating the X-rays after seven to ten days. Technetium bone scan will show up such fractures if this technology is available. More than one fracture showing on bone scans should lead to consideration of the possibility of child abuse.

If the history and X-rays do not suggest fracture, blood should be taken for blood count, sedimentation rate and culture to exclude the possibility of osteomyelitis or septic arthritis. Early diagnosis of septic arthritis is crucial since irreversible damage to articular cartilage can occur very rapidly. Diagnostic joint aspiration under general anaesthetic is indicated where septic arthritis is suspected. Technetium bone scanning may be used to confirm localised infection. Treatment for suspected osteomyelitis or septic arthritis should be instituted if the clinical features (i.e. local tenderness, evidence of joint pain, systemic upset) in combination with elevated white cell count or ESR suggest the diagnosis. Treatment must be given initially by the intravenous route with antibiotics such as flucloxacillin and fucidic acid.

Older children

The history is generally more helpful and will narrow down the differential diagnosis more faithfully than in toddlers. Remember, in all age groups – hip pain may present as pain anywhere from the hip to the knee. Examination of the hip is as for toddlers. In peripubertal patients, hip symptomatology would suggest the possibility of slipped upper femoral epiphysis, which is frequently bilateral even if the contralateral side is asymptomatic. These patients are frequently overweight and the diagnosis is important to expedite internal fixation preventing further slippage and resultant ischaemic damage to the femoral head.

Situations of 'No diagnosis'

Where the history is non-specific and there are no abnormal signs, normal blood tests and X-rays it is worth deferring further investigation for five to six days and reviewing if the limp is persistent. Advise parents to return sooner if the symptoms deteriorate or the child becomes systemically unwell. In the majority of cases these patients' symptoms disappear and one is left with a retrospective diagnosis of 'soft tissue injury'.

Key points

- Observation provides the most helpful clinical information.
- Fever, pseudoparesis and local pain is due to osteomyelitis until proven otherwise.
- Septic arthritis must be diagnosed and treated promptly to prevent joint damage.

14 Oedema

Introduction

Oedema is caused by excessive interstitial fluid. It may be localised or generalised, pitting or non-pitting. Excessive tissue fluid can accumulate as a result of transudation where capillary oncotic pressure is low (usually due to hypoproteinaemia), or exudation where there is an inflammatory process. The clinical assessment should enable one to decide whether the problem is local or general, exudative or transudative and if transudative, whether the problem is renal, intestinal or hepatic.

Clinical evaluation

History

Parents will rarely present with 'oedema' as a symptom. They are more likely to notice local or generalised swelling. Define the onset, distribution and severity of the symptom. Enquire as to whether there are any concomitant symptoms such as fever, skin rash, stridor or pain. Specifically enquire as to the presence of symptoms that would indicate cardiac, renal, hepatic, or intestinal pathology.

Clinical examination

Where there is oedema present see if this is pitting in nature. Non-pitting oedema suggests a chronic problem involving the lymphatics or associated with denervation. Check the vital signs – hypoproteinaemic oedema may be associated with significant volume depletion and consequent signs of hypovolaemia. The temperature may be elevated if there is an inflammatory cause. Look for any evidence of chronic liver disease such as spider naevi or visible veins on the anterior abdominal wall. When examining the cardiovascular system check for the presence of a pericardial effusion. In examining the chest percuss the bases carefully to detect pleural effusions. Examination of the abdomen should include an evaluation of liver size and consistency; also check for splenomegaly which may imply the presence of portal hypertension. Where oedema is present this commonly affects the genitalia particularly when the child is ambulant. Check carefully for the presence of ascites and measure the abdominal circumference.

Measurement of height, weight and nutritional indices are important but may be difficult to interpret where there is severe ascites. In these cases observation is important in assessing nutrition – look carefully at the axilla for evidence of subcutaneous fat loss. In advanced nephrotic syndrome there may be additional complications, such as peritonitis or deep venous thrombosis.

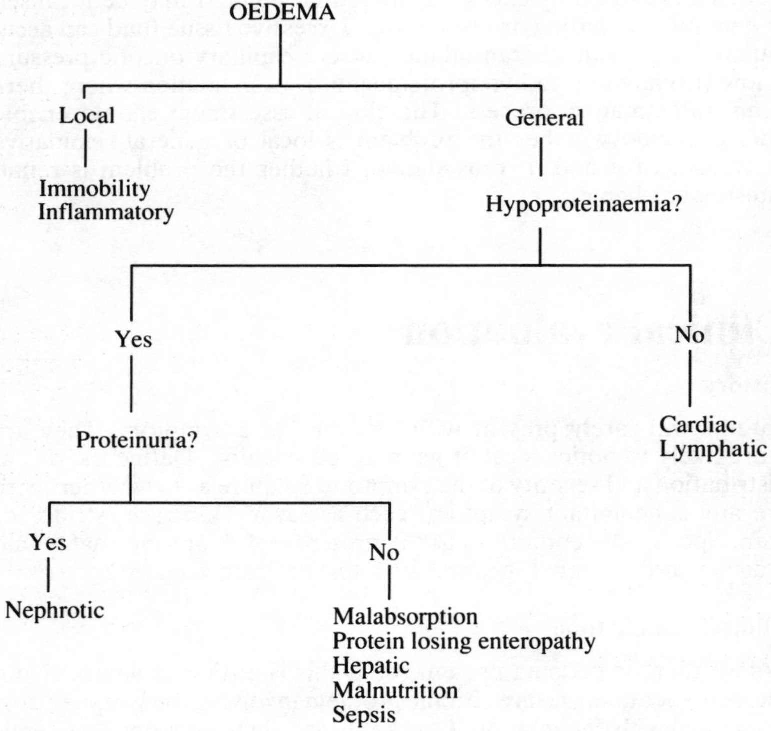

Fig. 14.1 Diagnostic pathway for assessment of oedema

Diagnosis

The major investigative and diagnostic decisions depend on three pieces of information:

1. Is this a local or general condition?
2. If generalised, is there hypoproteinaemia?
3. If there is hypoproteinaemia is there proteinuria?

Local oedema

Where local oedema occurs acutely it may be part of an allergic response, i.e. angio-oedema. In this case, onset is rapid following contact with an allergen and there are usually other symptoms such as itching, skin rash, stridor and possible tachycardia. This condition can evolve to full-blown anaphylaxis upon repeated exposure. Management is directed towards finding the cause of the symptom complex and treatment with antihistamines, and in severe cases adrenaline and hydrocortisone. Local inflammation associated with infection or vasculitis can also give rise to oedema. Where there is infection the child is usually febrile and toxic and there will usually be other signs such as heat and tenderness. Henoch–Schonlein purpura can cause local oedema particularly on the feet and scalp. Chronic denervation and immobility may be associated with local oedema, usually of the lower limb.

Generalised oedema

Generalised oedema is usually first noted on the face when the child wakes in the morning. As the day proceeds facial oedema diminishes but scrotal and lower limb oedema then become apparent. The child may have few or no symptoms until the process is quite advanced. In evaluating generalised oedema it is necessary to decide whether the problem is associated with hypoproteinaemia. Where the serum albumin level is normal this would suggest that the oedema is associated with a lymphatic or a cardiac problem. Congestive heart failure causing oedema is exceedingly rare in childhood but may be found with constrictive pericardiasis or cor pulmonale. Generalised oedema associated with lymphatic pathology is rare and usually hereditary.

Hypoproteinaemia

Hypoproteinaemia can be due to malabsorption, failure of synthesis or excessive protein loss in the urine or the gut.

Malabsorption Hypoproteinaemic oedema may occur as a consequence of cystic fibrosis, coeliac disease, or any of the other malabsorptive states. In these conditions oedema is rarely the major presenting symptom.

Synthetic failure This usually implies advanced hepatic disease. Where hepatic dysfunction has led to ascites, there is invariably some element of portal hypertension. The investigation and management will depend on the other features present. Oedema and ascites in isolation, rarely give rise to symptoms and it is important that overenthusiastic treatment of these signs does not compromise the child's well-being.

Protein losing enteropathies These can rarely cause hypoproteinaemia. Where there are overt signs of inflammatory bowel disease, diagnosis may be straightforward but in marginal cases detailed studies of protein loss in stool are indicated.

Renal loss of albumin Loss must be significant, e.g. more than 2 g per 24 hours, before the hepatic compensatory mechanisms are overcome and hypoproteinaemia occurs. In children with significant proteinuria the major decision is whether this is due to minimal change glomerular nephritis or more serious pathology. If the child is under five years of age, the blood pressure, urea and creatinine levels are normal, the proteinuria selective and not associated with haematuria, it is very likely that minimal change glomerular nephritis is responsible. Where this is the case empiric treatment with prednisolone is indicated. If there are atypical features this would suggest the possibility of alternative pathologies such as SLE or mesangio-capillary glomerular nephritis. In these instances, evaluation by a specialist paediatric nephrologist is indicated.

Key points

- Always test urine for proteinuria.
- Hypoproteinuria can be due to inadequate intake, failure of synthesis, or loss in the gut, urine or extravascular space.
- Minimal change of glomerulonephritis occurs in preschool children, who have normal blood pressure, renal function, complement levels, whose proteinuria is selective, and who do not have haematuria.

Useful literature

- Oedema, S. Osofsky and J.E. Lewy. In: *Clinical paediatric nephrology*, R. Postlethwaite (ed.) (Wright, 1986)

15 Poisoning

Introduction

Poisoning in childhood can be considered under two main age groups: preschool toddlers and teenagers. In toddlers poisoning is generally accidental, occurs at home and presents rapidly for medical attention.

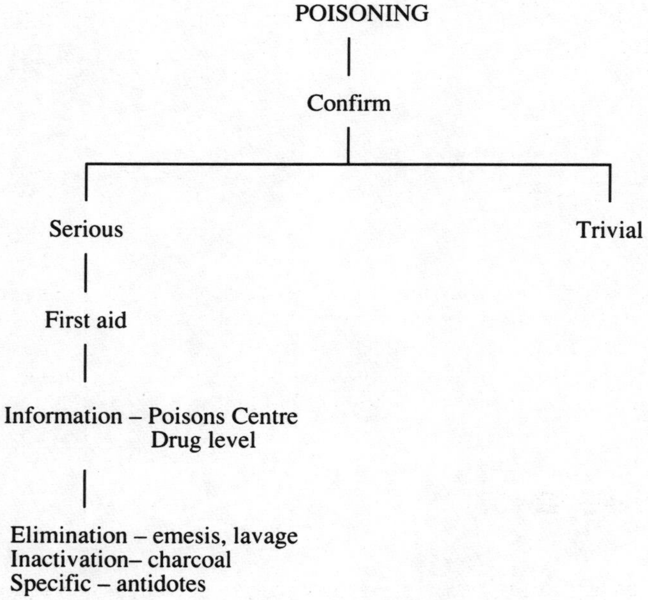

Fig. 15.1 Pathway for management of suspected poisoning

Approximately half the incidents involve the ingestion of materials normally found in the home such as cleaning agents, cosmetics and cooking materials. The remainder involve medicinal preparations. The prognosis is usually good.

In the teenage group poisonings are frequently intentional. Medicines are generally involved, household compounds rarely. There may be a delay in seeking medical attention. The poisoning is more likely to cause significant morbidity than in toddlers. Very rarely poisoning in young infants may occur as part of 'Munchausen's syndrome by proxy' (Meadow syndrome). In these cases the history is usually withheld and the diagnostic challenge is uncovering that poisoning has occurred.

History

In most cases children will present accompanied by parents with a history of accidental ingestion of some product or drug. The parents may be unsure as to the quantity consumed or indeed as to the nature of the medication taken. Try to establish clearly exactly what was taken, when, and how much (expressed in milligrams per kilogram). Drug ingestions may be multiple. If the parents have not brought a sample with them, send one home to bring back a sample of the drug and, if possible, the container.

Examination

The urgency of the initial sequence of events will be determined by the clinical condition of the child and by the nature of the ingested compounds. Where the child has collapsed initial resuscitation should proceed. Establish baseline vital signs and level of consciousness. Document any unusual neurological behaviour.

Management

Initial resuscitation, when necessary, requires attention to the ABC of resuscitation, i.e. airway patency, breathing efficacy and gas exchange, circulatory integrity.

Airway

Children whose level of consciousness has been impaired by tranquillising medication may have suppression of airway protective reflexes. Induced vomiting is especially dangerous in such patients and is contraindicated. If these children do vomit, they should be placed in the left lateral, head down position and suction of the oropharynx and nasopharynx carried out immediately. If emptying the stomach is indicated this should be done with the use of a wide-bore orogastric tube with prior tracheal intubation to secure the airway. Caustic acid and alkalis can be particularly dangerous in this situation.

Breathing

Tranquillisers in overdosage may depress respiration. Any child with an impaired level of consciousness should have a careful assessment made of ventilatory effort. Oxygen should be administered. If ventilatory effort is insufficient, bag and mask ventilation will be necessary. Specific antidotes such as naloxone may be of value; if not, endotracheal intubation and mechanical ventilation should proceed.

Circulation

This should be assessed with standard methods of pulse, blood pressure and capillary filling time. Where there is hypovolaemia an initial bolus of plasma, saline or 5 per cent albumin – 10 ml/kg – should be given.

Emptying the stomach and preventing further absorption

Syrup of ipecacuanha is an effective, safe, locally and centrally acting emetic. Dosages of 15 ml in children under 5 years and 30 ml in those over should be followed by a drink of water. If there is no vomiting within 15 minutes, repeat the dose. It is contraindicated where there is a lowered level of consciousness, absent gag reflex or where caustics or petroleum extracts have been taken. Ipecac induces compulsive, powerful vomiting, which is very unpleasant for the patient. There is a tendency to give this to all children who have been accidentally poisoned and present to hospital. This may not be necessary and one should always check first whether the compound ingested is indeed harmful before causing unnecessary and unpleasant vomiting.

Activated charcoal is much underused in the initial management of ingestions because of the work required to administer it. Charcoal binds drugs to its huge adsorptive surface area, rendering them unavailable for absorption into the bloodstream. It is pharmacologically inactive itself. It adsorbs most drugs effectively with a varying degree of affinity. Charcoal is ineffective with metals, alcohols, boric acid, mineral acids, caustic alkalis, malathion, cyanide and DDT. Charcoal should be administered in an iced water slurry. This preparation is very messy – so wear an apron! Never give with milk or ice cream. A dosage of approximately eight to ten times the ingested amounts of drug should be given, 10–30 grams is a practical choice. Repeated doses over a 48 hour period may be indicated following admission to hospital in situations where a drug with enterohepatic circulation has been taken, e.g. digoxin, tricyclic antidepressants. Charcoal traps these drugs as they are excreted in bile. Repeated doses may also be necessary if enteric coated or sustained release products have been taken. Sodium sulphate or magnesium sulphate should be given to expedite the passage of the drug/charcoal complex through the gut. A dosage of 250 mg/kg is appropriate for both these agents.

Ipecac may not be effective if large numbers of capsules or tablets form a 'chemical bezoar' in the stomach. This will be too big to be vomited and constitutes a pharmacological 'time bomb'. Where this is suspected endoscopy may be necessary to effect clearance. Repeated doses of activated charcoal are also useful in this instance to adsorb the drug being serially released by digestion of the chemical bezoar.

Generally, most ingested compounds will have emptied from the stomach within three hours of ingestion. However, some drugs which delay gastric emptying may persist for longer. These would include drugs with anticholinergic properties, particularly tricyclic antidepressants, opiates and atropine-like drugs. Do not give ipecac concomitantly with activated charcoal – the charcoal will adsorb the ipecac and prevent emesis and the ipecac will occupy the binding sites on the charcoal, rendering both ineffective.

Information

This lies at the heart of successful management of any specific poisoning. All acute paediatric services should have immediately at hand a comprehensive, up to date, text book on all poisoning. No one can be expected to remember the specific management of all drugs. Principles of management are important and one of the most important of these is to know where to get specific information. Regional, national and international centres specialising in toxicology are available at the end of a telephone.

Table 15.1 Frequently ingested products that are usually non-toxic

Abrasives
Adhesives
Antacids
Antibiotics
Baby product cosmetics
Ballpoint pen inks
Bathtub floating toys
Bath oil (castor oil & perfume)
Bleach (less than 6 per cent sodium hypochlorite)
Body conditioners
Bubble bath soaps (detergents)
Calamine lotion
Candles (beeswax or paraffin)
Caps (toy pistols, potassium chlorate)
Chalk (calcium carbonate)
Clay (modelling)
Colognes
Contraceptives
Corticosteroids
Cosmetics
Crayons (marked AP, CP)
Dehumidifying packets (silica or charcoal)
Detergents
Deodorants
Deodorizers (spray and refrigerator)
Etch-A-Sketch contents
Eye makeup
Fabric softeners
Fertilisers (if not insecticide or herbicides added)
Fish bowl additives
Glues and pastes
Golf ball (core may cause mechanical injury
Grease
Hair products (dyes may be caustic sprays, tonics)
Hand lotions and creams
Hydrogen peroxide (medicinal 3 per cent)
Incense
Indelible markers
Ink (black, blue – non permanent)
Idophil disinfectant
Laxatives
Lipstick
Lubricant
Lubricating oils (lipoid pneumonia)
Lysol brand disinfectant (not toilet bowl cleaner)
Magic Markers
Makeup (eye, liquid facial)
Matches
Mineral oil (unless aspirated)
Newspaper (chronic may result lead poisoning)
Paint, indoor, latex
Pencil (lead-graphite, colouring)
Perfumes
Petroleum jelly (Vaseline)
Phenophthalein laxatives (Ex-Lax)
Play-Doh
Polaroid picture coating fluid
Porous-tip ink marking pens
Prussian blue (ferricyanide)
Putty (less than 2 oz)
Rouge
Rubber cement
Sachets (essential oils, powder, talc aspiration)
Shampoos (liquid)
Shaving creams and lotions
Soap and soap products
Suntan preparation
Sweetening agents (saccharin, cyclamates)
Teething rings (water sterility)
Thermometers (mercury)
Thyroid tablet (dessicated)
Toilet water (alcohol)
Toothpaste (with or without fluoride)
Vaseline
Vitamins (with or without fluoride)
Warfarin (under 0.5 per cent)
Water colours
Zinc oxide
Zirconium oxide

Specific problems

- Caustic acid or alkali ingestions cause serious damage to the oesophagus and may result in oesophageal stricture. Usually there will be evidence of damage to the tongue and mouth, indicating further pathology lower down. Water should be given early and in large volumes to dilute the caustic in the oesophagus. Long-term follow-up by endoscopy is indicated where ingestion is serious.
- Phenothiazines and related drugs can result in an idiosyncratic acute dystonic state in children. Diphenhydramine 2.5–5 mg/kg dose intravenously reverses this effect immediately. Relapse may occur so that it is important to observe for at least 2 hours prior to discharge.
- Opiate-induced depression of consciousness and respiration may be reversed with naloxone in a dosage of 0.4–4 mg per dose IV. As with other antidotes, the effect wears off and the dose may need to be repeated.
- Paracetamol given in a toxic dose may result in delayed onset hepatic and renal problems. It is important to ascertain the dose ingested. The necessity of treatment with the antidote acetylcysteine can be calculated from measurement of the plasma level four hours after the ingestion.
- Where drugs and plants have atropine-like side effects physostigmine salicylate 0.5 mg IV is effective but may need to be given repeatedly.

This section has covered the initial steps in the management of acute poisonings. As with all childhood accidents, prevention is the key. Educational programmes for parents, legislation in the area of childproof drug containers and prohibition of the sale of dangerous compounds in accessible containers will be the most effective measures to prevent poisoning in children.

Key points

- Ipecac is overused.
- Charcoal is effective, but messy and underutilised.
- Agents which delay gastric emptying may be retrieved many hours after ingestion.
- Serious poisoning is rare.
- Always obtain guidance from the poisons centre – treatments can change!

Useful literature

- *Manual of emergency paediatrics*, 4th edition, R. Reece (W.B. Saunders, 1992)

16 Seizure

Introduction

Some 5 per cent of children have one or more seizures during childhood. For the parents, this is probably the most distressing event of their child's life. Many are convinced their child is dying but recovery brings the worry of recurrence or long-term sequelae. This emergency is one of the commonest, accounting for over 5 per cent of all paediatric hospitalisations. For a perspective, the likely causes of seizures are listed in Table 16.1 but in practice the majority are due to febrile convulsions. When the child presents, a calm efficient approach is necessary to effect rapid diagnosis and treatment and to reassure parents and attending staff. Diagnostic and therapeutic manoeuvres proceed together following loosely the pathway suggested in Figure 16.1. It is often helpful to delegate acute management to one physician, whilst another can record the history carefully.

Table 16.1 Cause of seizure

- Febrile convulsions
- Epilepsy
- Trauma
- CNS infections, inflammations
- Poisoning
- Metabolic disturbances
- Hypertension

Confirm

A rapid clinical appraisal, paying particular attention to vital signs, colour, muscle tone and level of consciousness, will usually allow confirmation that a seizure is present. Conditions which may be confused with seizure are listed on Table 16.2.

Classic seizure manifestations of tonic clonic movements, incontinence and tongue biting may be absent in early infancy where seizures may be more subtle. If seizures are very prolonged they may be associated with decerebrate posturing related to raised intracranial pressure.

Some patients with established medical conditions may have a Medic-alert bracelet indicating adrenal insufficiency or diabetes.

SEIZURE

↓

Confirm

↓

First aid

Check sugar

↓

Stop fit

Supportive

↓

Longterm — Treatment, Investigations, Parents

Fig. 15.1 Pathway for management of acute seizure

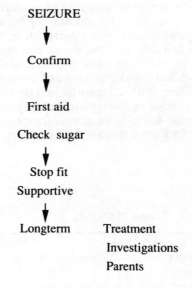

Table 16.2 Seizures may be confused with several entities, including the following

Symptom/sign	Distinction from seizure
Syncope	Bradycardia, pallor, hypotonia
Tetany	Carpopedal spasm, hyperventilation
Severe pain especially peritoneal	Vacant stare, episodic pallor
Rigor/fever	Delirium, consciousness retained
Drug-induced dystonia	Conscious, history of anti emetic ingestion
Benign sleep myoclonus	Movements abolished by postural or sleep state change
Shock	Hypovolaemia due to sepsis, adrenal crisis, dehydration
Arrhythmia	Bradycardia or tachycardia

First aid

Having confirmed the presence of a significant seizure, proceed with first aid along the A,B,C model:

Airway

Ensure that this is clear. Place the patient in the semiprone position.

Breathing

Check the patient's colour and check for good chest wall movement and breath sounds. Administer artificial respiration if indicated.

Circulation

Palpate pulses in the neck or the femorals to ensure an adequate pulse volume and heart rate.

At this stage it would also be important to check the blood sugar with a simple bedside stick test, as hypoglycaemia warrants the most rapid diagnosis. Next terminate the seizure. Where blood sugar is low give IV dextrose or SC glucagon; in the absence of hypoglycaemia treatment with diazepam is appropriate. This is most simply given rectally in a dose of 5 or 10 milligrams depending on the child's weight. Rectal diazepam will take about three minutes to work. If intravenous access is feasible, diazepam may be given intravenously in a dose of 0.25 milligrams per kilogram, slowly.

Clinical evaluation

Obtain a careful history of the seizure from a witness. Pay particular attention to any preceding events, the precise description of the patient's movements as the seizure evolved and the duration of seizure. It is important to ascertain whether the patient is taking any medication.

In the past history ask about perinatal events, immunisation and developmental history and also any previous history of seizures. Previous hospitalisations for severe illness or head injury are also important. Social history will provide important clues as to contact with infectious diseases, the possibility of accidental drug ingestion or indeed a background to suggest the possibility of non-accidental injury. There may be a family history of seizures or inherited metabolic and neurodegenerative conditions.

Clinical examination

On occasion the smell from the patient's breath will provide useful clues to ketosis, metabolic derangement or drug ingestion. Measurement of the child's weight is vital for calculation of drug and fluid prescriptions. Head circumference may reveal aetiological factors such as micro-, macro- or hydrocephalus. Palpate for the presence of ventriculoperitoneal shunt. Measurement of the vital signs is important to provide baseline information and also to detect clues as to seizure aetiology. Pay particular attention to measurement of blood pressure. Assess the patient's oxygenation and if available, measure the oxygen saturation.

Neurological examination is clearly the most important but may be clouded by postictal drowsiness or the effect of anticonvulsant drugs. Document the level of consciousness and pupillary reactions. Check the fundi for signs of papilloedema or haemorrhage. Test for meningism and do a full neurological examination though this will almost certainly need to be repeated when the patient has recovered from the effect of seizure. Look for signs of aspiration in the respiratory system. Examine the abdomen carefully, paying particular attention to enlargement of the liver, spleen or kidneys and looking for any unusual masses.

A skin rash may give clues to the aetiology. A petechial rash could be due to meningococcal sepsis, or thrombocytopenia. 'Neuro' cutaneous syndromes such as neurofibromatosis, Sturge–Weber syndrome and incontinentia pigmenti have characteristic rashes. Scald encephalopathy is a possibility where burns, even trivial, are present. Where fever is present check for foci in the ears and throat.

Laboratory evaluation

Since the differential diagnosis of an acute seizure is bewilderingly long, clearly it is necessary to be selective in laboratory evaluation. The relevance of particular investigations will depend on the clinical assessment, in particular the severity of the seizure, the response to anticonvulsants and the degree of illness. It is useful to think through the various divisions of the pathology department and to assess whether individual investigations are relevant. The more urgent and commonly indicated tests are discussed first.

Biochemistry

Measurement of blood sugar is especially important and should be undertaken at the bed side at the initial evaluation. Hypoglycaemia may be the primary cause of seizures in a treated diabetic or in ketotic hypoglycaemia. In addition it may indicate Reye's syndrome, inborn error of metabolism or evolving hepatic failure. A prolonged seizure may give rise to secondary hypoglycaemia which will aggravate the neurological injury. An elevated blood sugar is a frequent finding in the aftermath of a seizure and probably reflects an adrenal 'stress' response.

The blood urea may be elevated in dehydration or in renal failure, particularly haemolytic uraemic syndrome. Very low blood urea is sometimes associated with hepatic failure. The presence of a normal urea does not exclude significant dehydration. Disturbances of sodium balance resulting in hyper- or hyponatraemia may trigger seizures. The potassium level may be elevated in established renal failure but is rarely implicated in the aetiology of seizure. Hypocalcaemia associated with hypoparathryoidism or inappropriate infant feeding may cause seizure. The serum calcium level may also be depressed in severe illness as a non-specific finding. Hypercalcaemia rarely causes seizures. Hypomagnesaemia is usually associated with malabsorption and may cause tetany or seizures.

Measurement of hepatic transaminases and blood ammonia are important if Reye's syndrome is suspected. The bilirubin level may be elevated if there is haemolysis as in haemolytic-uraemic syndrome but is usually normal in Reye's syndrome. Blood gas should be measured if there is any doubt regarding oxygenation or if metabolic causes are suspected. The finding of the metabolic acidosis in the absence of an obvious cause (e.g. dehydration) would suggest the possibility of organic acidaemia. A sample of urine should be taken for measurement of amino acids and snap frozen in liquid nitrogen for organic acids assay if the clinical situation suggests an inborn error of metabolism. Blood levels of anticonvulsants should be measured, if relevant, to allow differentiation between non-compliance and poor drug efficacy.

Haematology

A full blood count is ordered reflexively in most acute situations. Low haemoglobin may indicate anaemia associated with infection or microangiopathic haemolysis. A high white cell count may be an indicator of bacterial sepsis or may simply be a stress response following a seizure. The platelet count will be depressed in thrombocytopenic purpura and in disseminated intravascular coagulation. A blood film may indicate parasitic disease, haemoglobinopathy or haemolysis. A precise differential white cell count will give a more accurate indication of whether bacterial sepsis is a problem and a film may give clues as to the presence of lead poisoning. Tests of blood coagulation will be indicated if a bleeding cause or liver dysfunction is suspected. The ESR is a non-specific indicator of inflammation and rarely advances a specific diagnosis.

Microbiology

If the child presents with a febrile convulsion it is important to exclude serious underlying infection. If a focus is not apparent on clinical examination, urine and blood should be cultured. The place of CSF examination is controversial. Since clinical diagnosis of meningitis in infancy is difficult, some authorities recommend that all children under 1 year presenting with a febrile convulsion should have a lumbar puncture. Caution is advisable, however, since lumbar puncture, in the presence of septicaemia, may increase the risk of meningitis and in the presence of established cerebral oedema, may cause coning. Lumbar puncture of the vigorous child is frequently traumatic and does not provide diagnostic information. A helpful indicator is that 'positive' lumbar punctures are usually easy; the vigorous, mobile infant is unlikely to have turbid CSF. Viral cultures may be taken;

where relevant, antibody measurement will assist a retrospective diagnosis of certain virus and bacterial infections. Electron microscopy of vesicles may indicate herpetic infection.

Imaging

A chest X-ray may be indicated if pneumonia or aspiration is suspected. Skull X-ray generally has a low yield but may indicate a fracture or intracranial calcification. CT scan is rarely indicated but may be helpful if parenchymal lesions, intracranial haemorrhage or herpetic encephalitis is suspected.

Other tests

Electroencephalography will usually be abnormal in the postictal state and as such, the diagnostic and prognostic information provided is of limited value. Nevertheless it may help support the diagnosis of hypsarrhythmia or encephalitis. Electrocardiorgraphy with 24 hour monitoring may be indicated if arrhythmia is suspected.

Management

Anticonvulsant

Diazepam in a dosage of 0.25 milligrams per kilogram IV is the drug of choice. The dose may be repeated if necessary. Paraldehyde intramuscularly is an alternative to diazepam. Should seizure persist despite serial doses of diazepam, consideration should be given to an additional anticonvulsant. Phenobarbitone has long been a tried and trusted anticonvulsant but it is now falling into disrepute largely because of its relatively poor efficacy and side effects in long-term usage. Phenytoin is a useful agent but administration may cause cardiac side effects and necessitates regular monitoring of plasma levels. Intravenous sodium valproate is a further option though experience with this preparation is limited.

Should seizure persist despite further anticonvulsants the possibility of raised intracranial pressure should be considered. This may be evident clinically as decerebrate posturing. In these circumstances an infusion of mannitol may restore sensitivity to anticonvulsant medication.

Should the seizure persist for more than one hour, transfer the patient to an intensive care unit and consider sedation, paralysis and ventilation. Under continuous EEG control, thiopentone is undoubtedly the most potent anticonvulsant but may be associated with severe side effects such as hypotension. When the seizure has been controlled a decision regarding long-term treatment is needed.

Supportive measures

If the child is febrile ensure that hydration is adequate and that excess clothing has been removed. Paracetamol may be given orally or rectally and if fever persists, sponging with tepid water is helpful. It is important that cold water or direct fanning is not used since these both result in peripheral vasoconstriction with a consequent, paradoxical, further increase in core temperature.

Metabolic balance may be assessed by clinical and laboratory methods. If hypernatraemia is present it is important to correct this slowly. Hypoglycaemia may be an ongoing problem if there is liver dysfunction and infusions of hypertonic dextrose may be necessary. Monitoring of fluid output is important since early peritoneal dialysis would be indicated in some cases of haemolytic uraemic syndrome.

Raised intracranial pressure

The possibility of intracranial hypertension should be entertained if the patient's seizures are refractory or if the level of consciousness remains impaired. Simple clinical measurements of pulse, blood pressure, pupillary reaction and fundoscopy appearances will help. If the patient remains comatose with suggestive clinical signs, intracranial pressure should probably be monitored directly. Insertion of a subarachnoid bolt or a ventricular catheter is a specialist procedure and best undertaken by an experienced neurosurgeon.

Direct measurement of intracranial pressure and arterial blood pressure will allow the calculation of the cerebral perfusion pressure which is the most important indicator of neural well-being. Blood pressure may need to be supported with inotropes. If intracranial pressure rises, it may be lowered with mannitol, hyperventilation, direct CSF drainage and in rare instances by direct decompression by a craniotomy.

Parents

Even where the seizure is terminated abruptly, parents will take some time to recover. If the child has ongoing problems the parents' distress will be severe. It is important to make time to sit and explain developments to the parents and, moreover, to listen.

Specific

If an underlying infection is detected then antibiotic treatment is indicated. Where encephalitis is suspected clinically it may be possible to have direct virological confirmation or supporting evidence from EEG and CT. Acyclovir is active against herpetic encephalitis and will probably diminish mortality though morbidity remains a problem. Where meningitis is established antibiotic treatment should proceed along conventional lines. Consideration should be given to treatment with dexamethasone, administered before the antibiotics, particularly if *Haemophilus influenzae* is implicated. This approach may reduce the incidence of sequelae including deafness. Regular monitoring of head circumference (subdural effusion) and fluid balance (inappropriate ADH secretion) are appropriate.

Further investigation

Detailed metabolic studies involving protein loading and response to various physiological stresses may be indicated if complex metabolic problems are suspected.

Key points

- Always check the blood sugar.
- Diazepam rectally or intravenously is the drug of choice.
- Talk to the parents, listen to the parents.

Useful literature

- *Paediatric neurology*, 2nd edition, E. Brett (Churchill Livingstone, 1991)

17 Sudden infant death/ apparent life-threatening event

Sudden infant death

Between the ages of one and 12 months, about five babies per thousand will die. Approximately half of these deaths are unexpected.

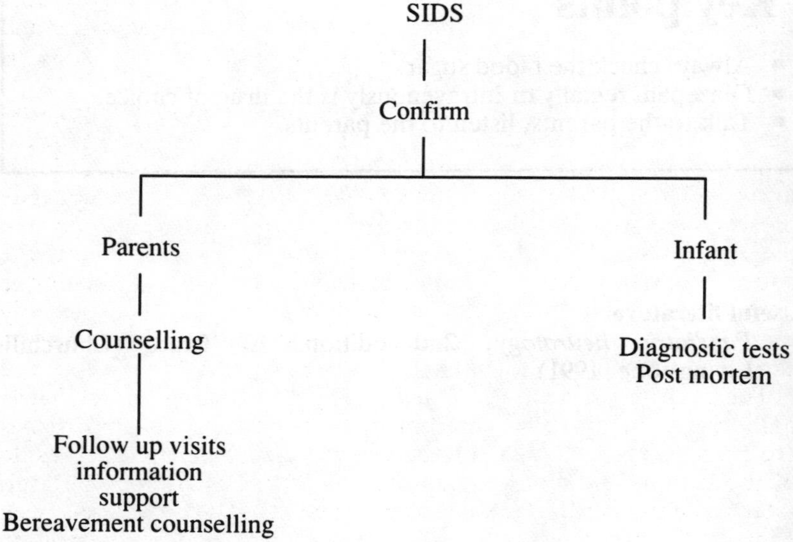

Fig. 17.1 Management pathway for SIDS

In most cases these unexpected deaths remain unexplained even after a detailed post mortem examination – sudden infant death syndrome (SIDS). Sudden, unexpected death may also be caused by overwhelming infection, inborn errors of metabolism, myocarditis or undiagnosed congenital malformations. Where sudden unexpected death has occurred the role of the doctor is to confirm the death or provide resuscitation where this is appropriate, to try to establish a diagnosis, particularly if this has genetic implications, and to provide psychological first aid and ongoing support to the bereaved family.

Management

The child is likely to be discovered at home and parents may rush to hospital without giving any advance warning. When called to a possible SIDS victim it is important to remain calm but efficient – 'the first procedure at a cardiac arrest is to take your own pulse'. The fact of death first needs to be established. If there is doubt, however, and if resuscitation is attempted, a senior doctor should be involved immediately. Relatives of the infant should be informed of the fact of death as soon as possible in a sensitive manner, out of the public eye. Though it may prove difficult, it is important to obtain an adequate history. This should include the circumstances in which the infant was found, sleeping position, the amount of clothing and any suggestion of infection prior to death. The past history should clearly document complications of pregnancy, parental smoking and any adverse perinatal history. Family history of previous SIDS or apparent life-threatening event (ALTE) should be sought.

The initial physical examination should document rectal temperature, state of nutrition and growth. Look for any signs of external bruising, abrasions, petechiae or fractures. Obtain cultures of blood, urine and CSF to seek infectious causes of the child's death. The presence of hypostatic discoloration will depend on the time between the infant's death and discovery; its pattern will corroborate the baby's terminal position. In most cases the physical examination is unremarkable. As the infant has died suddenly and unexpectedly there will need to be an inquest and a post mortem. This must be explained tactfully to the parents.

The necropsy should be carried out by an experienced paediatric pathologist. In up to 80 per cent of cases petechial haemorrhages are present, typically beneath the visceral pleura, under the capsule of the thymus and along the coronary arteries. There may be aspirated vomitus in the larger airways. The lungs are generally well expanded. Histology tends to be non-specific, showing pulmonary congestion and oedema, with possibly some mild inflammation of the upper airways. Bacterial cultures are often unhelpful and may cause problems in interpretation since post mortem contamination is common.

Parents

As indicated earlier, when the fact of death is established the parents are informed. It is very difficult for parents to come to terms with sudden infant death. Death is sudden and unexpected, leaving no opportunity for anticipatory grief. There is often no definite cause, so parents find it difficult to rationalise the death. The death may have occurred shortly after the mother went back to work outside the home or shortly after the infant was moved out of the parents' bedroom. This can add major guilt and self-blame.

Counselling should begin with a sensitive and thoughtful approach as soon as the baby is seen. Informing parents of the fact of death must be done with a lot of empathy. Parents should be allowed as much time as they want with their baby, away from other people. It can be helpful if photographs are taken; at a later stage these will help establish the reality of death. In explaining the requirement for an autopsy the parents must be reassured that this will be carried out sensitively, that the family will be able to see the baby after the examination and the preliminary results will be available within two days. Siblings should be encouraged to see the baby and to be present at the funeral. Staff should be able to advise parents regarding local funeral arrangements. The family doctor, community nurse and local clergy should also be informed.

An appointment should be made with an appropriate person, preferably a senior paediatrician, for about two weeks after the death. The purpose of this meeting is to give complete post mortem results, to answer the numerous questions that parents will have, to assess how they and their other children are coping and to advise them about the likely course of grief. This should include explaining differences between grief of father and mother and the importance of catharsis. Many people have difficulty in talking about a child's death. This may result in their friends either avoiding them or talking about anything other than the death of the baby. It is important to be aware that very little will be remembered of the initial visit and that all relevant information may need to be reiterated on a number of occasions. Subsequent visits should be arranged 6 to 8 weeks later and further appointments depending on the progress of the grief. It is not necessary that bereavement counsellors be involved in the majority of cases but there should be 'more thought, sensitivity, and activity on the part of existing professional groups'.

Parents may be very concerned about the possibility of recurrence. If there have been any obvious risk factors – for instance, maternal smoking, overwrapping or prone sleeping position – advice regarding these should be given in a way that will avoid self-blame. Arrangements should be made for a full examination of subsequent infants and in some instances parents are happier if an apnoea monitor is supplied.

Monitoring

The recommendation that infants at risk of sudden infant death syndrome should be monitored assumes that firstly, at-risk groups can be identified and secondly, that monitors will give sufficient time for resuscitation to be carried out.

The known risk factors for SIDS are not specific or sensitive enough to identify the infants who will need monitoring. Nor is there any proof that reversible apnoea precedes reversible brain injury or indeed that apnoea monitors have any impact on SIDS. Nevertheless there is often strong parental and professional pressure for their use.

The commonly used monitors are respiratory monitors, generally using a pressure pad. These will detect central apnoea where respiratory effort has stopped. They may fail to alarm if activated by body movements and also in some cases of obstructive apnoea. More sophisticated monitoring would include pulse oximetry and transcutaneous oxygen monitors. The role of this form of monitoring is still controversial but can certainly provide useful insights on a research basis.

In spite of these limitations, some families who have had a sudden infant death or an apparent life-threatening event are less anxious where a monitor is provided. In any situation where an apnoea monitor is recommended the carers must be given instructions in the basic methods of cardiopulmonary resuscitation and they will also require ongoing emotional and technical support.

Aetiology of sudden infant death

By definition sudden infant death syndrome is unexplained. It is important, however, in the evaluation to try to establish whether there is an underlying explanation, particularly as this may have genetic implications. The most important group in this regard would be metabolic conditions such as medium chain acyl co-enzyme A dehydrogenase deficiency (MCAD) and glycogen storage diseases. Unfortunately these conditions may not always produce specific features on post mortem but their presence should be suspected if there is a family history or if there is microvesicular fatty change in the liver. Screening of subsequent siblings where there is any suggestion of a metabolic condition is important. The nature of investigation should be discussed with a specialist in metabolic medicine.

Infanticide is a contentious and controversial issue. Some authorities feel that up to 10 per cent of sudden infant deaths are due to infanticide and understandably parents' support groups and many professionals find this offensive. Infanticide should be suspected where the condition has recurred within a family, at an unusual age, or if there are major psychosocial stresses.

There are many other risk factors for sudden infant death. Based on epidemiological work it has recently been recommended that infants sleep on their backs or side, with a reduction in the amount of bedding used. Introduction of these guidelines appears to have caused a halving of the incidence of sudden infant death syndrome and future trends will be watched with interest. Maternal smoking is associated with an increased incidence of SIDS, and its effect is dose-related. It also increases the risk of respiratory illness in infants and children. For these reasons alone, cessation is recommended. Breastfeeding is also recommended – there is no evidence that it protects against SIDS, but it does diminish the risk of respiratory infection.

Key points

- Involve a senior colleague.
- Handle parents with compassion and patience.
- Allow parents to spend time with the dead infant, alone.
- Arrange follow-up for counselling and information exchange.

Useful literature

- Symposium on SIDS, A. Busuttil A, Burchell and A. Burchell (eds) (*Journal of clinical pathology., vol. 45, 1992).*

Apparent life-threatening event

Introduction

These episodes were previously called 'near-miss SIDS'. This terminology has been abandoned as it implies that SIDS may be averted, which may provoke unnecessary distress in affected parents, and the relationship between ALTE and SIDS remains unclear. ALTE is an episode in which an infant is found apnoeic, pale or cyanosed, and hypotonic, requiring vigorous resuscitation before breathing or movement is re-established. Most parents think that their infant would have died unless discovered. Since the parents are likely to be frightened the accuracy of their observations may be in some doubt. A number of these episodes are merely periodic breathing which is common during deep sleep especially in premature infants. Some apnoeic episodes are associated with pertussis and bronchiolitis. Infants who have sustained an ALTE have a 1–2 per cent risk of subsequent sudden infant death. There have been numerous studies of infants in this group with no consistent results.

History

It may be difficult to get an accurate history as the parents will be extremely frightened when they discover their infant apparently *in extremis*. It is very important, however, to clarify the events as much as possible because subsequent investigation and management will be influenced by the history. The history should document the child's well-being in the days prior to the event and a full pregnancy and birth history should be obtained. Enquire specifically for any history of vomiting suggesting gastro-oesophageal reflux. Previous episodes of pallor, sweating or tachypnoea may point towards cardiac dysrhythmia. History of immunisations and recent contact with infectious diseases should be sought. Some drugs, such as dicyclomine, may cause apnoea. A family history of ALTE or SIDS is important.

Evaluation

A complete physical, neurological and developmental examination is performed. Look for any abnormal bruising or abrasions. Further investigations can be carried out if it is decided that the episode was a true ALTE and not an over-reaction by the carer to a non-life-threatening event.

Full blood count, ESR, biochemistry and blood gas will indicate whether there is infection or metabolic abnormality. Where appropriate, blood, urine and CSF cultures should be taken. An ECG should be carried out to look for any abnormalities of rhythm and specifically prolonged QT interval which may be associated with sudden death. Twenty-four hour cardio-respiratory monitoring may give some clues as to abnormal breathing pattern and may also provide reassurance for parents and doctors. If there is any suspicion of gastro-oesophageal reflux a barium swallow and oesophageal pH monitoring should be performed. An EEG may be indicated as these episodes may be manifestations of seizures.

Subsequent management

There is at present no way of identifying the small number of ALTE infants who will subsequently die from SIDS. However, most parents are reassured by follow-up visits, the frequency depending on parental anxiety and abnormal findings. The question of apnoea monitoring has already been discussed.

Key points

- Investigate for infection, seizure or apnoea.
- Apnoea monitors do not prevent SIDS.

Useful literature

- Clinical presentation and management of near-miss S.I.D.S., Dunne K.P., Matthews T.G. (*Pediatrics* 1987, 79, 889–93)

18 Stridor

Introduction

Stridor is the sound of obstructed inspiration. It represents a local or segmental narrowing of the mid-airway, anywhere from the epiglottis down to the carina. If the narrowing is minimal, stridor will be present only when inspiratory airflow is increased, i.e. during rapid inspiration as in an anxious or crying child. The worse the narrowing, the

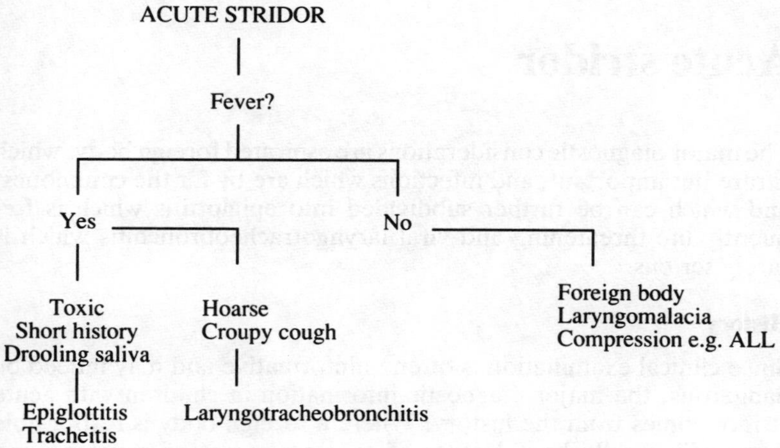

Fig. 18.1 Diagnostic pathway for acute stridor. If epiglottitis is suspected, the diagnosis should be confirmed and the airway secured by an experienced anaesthetist.

more constant the stridor, i.e. stridor during quiet inspiration. With severe narrowing inspiration is only achieved at the peak of negative intrathoracic pressure. In such cases a highpitched squeaking stridor represents all of inspiration and total occlusion is imminent.

In general stridor can be divided into chronic, which is usually due to congenital abnormalities, or acute which is usually due to infection or a foreign body.

Congenital stridor

Some infants have stridor from, or soon after, birth. The commonest reason for this is laryngomalacia. This is due to a laxity of the supporting tissues of the larynx and is a self-limiting condition usually resolving in the first year. Although most children with this abnormality thrive, occasionally where symptoms are severe it may lead to feeding difficulties and present with a failure to thrive. In such cases a laryngoscopy may be indicated to exclude other rarer causes such as tracheal stenosis, laryngeal malformations or, in the previously intubated infant, subglottic stenosis. Barium swallow may be necessary to exclude the possibility of a vascular ring.

Acute stridor

The major diagnostic considerations are aspirated foreign body, which is rare but important, and infections which are by far the commonest and which can be further subdivided into epiglottitis which is frequently life-threatening and viral laryngotracheobronchitis which is rarely serious.

History

Since clinical examination is often uninformative and may indeed be dangerous, the major diagnostic information in children with acute stridor comes from the history. Where a foreign body is responsible there will usually be a history of an acute onset of coughing and choking in the suggestive environment, e.g. peanut eating at a children's party. The rapidity of the onset of the stridor in the absence of signs of infection is very suggestive.

Though massive tonsillar enlargement or tonsillar abcess can cause stridor, for practical purposes it is infection at the level of the epiglottis, larynx and trachea which threatens patency of the airway. Epiglottitis occurs as part of a septicaemic illness due to *Haemophilus influenzae* type B. The normally flap shaped epiglottis swells up to a spherical shape and impinges upon the airway. Children of all ages are at risk though cases are commoner amongst preschool children. The history is characteristic. Symptoms are rapidly progressive over a 12 to 24 hour period. Children are pyrexial with signs of systemic toxicity. There is very marked stridor, drooling of saliva, dysphagia and a rather muffled speech pattern. Children are very reluctant to speak and they frequency assume unusual postures in an attempt to maximise the calibre of their already narrowed airway. These desperately held postures indicate a severely compromised airway. Children with epiglottitis will rarely have a cough.

Bacterial tracheitis is less common than epiglottitis and is characterised by a pyosanguinous infection of the mucosa of the trachea, gradually occluding the lumen. Symptoms, signs and initial management are similar to those for epiglottitis. Viral laryngotracheobronchitis may be caused by a variety of respiratory viruses and involves predominantly the larynx. It occurs most frequently in children under 2 years of age. The resultant oedema of the larynx and trachea results in the typical symptoms and signs. Progression to complete occlusion is rare. The onset is usually subacute and children may have been symptomatic for days prior to presentation. Symptoms are characteristically worse at night. Children have a very prominent dry 'croupy' cough and their voice and cry is typically hoarse. Stridor may be intermittent and most noticeable when the child cries or is agitated. Children are rarely toxic or systemically ill and pyrexia is usually only moderate or low grade. There is no dysphagia or drooling.

Examination

Where epiglottitis or foreign body is suspected from the history, examination should be limited to inspection from the end of the bed. In children with acute viral illness it is important to document the severity of the recession, whether present at rest, and the child's vital signs.

Management

Foreign body

Do not inspect the pharynx as this may cause gagging and precipitate acute blockage. Do not perform the Heimlich manoeuvre or the 'interscapular thump' unless a stable situation of partial obstruction acutely changes to complete occlusion. Thumping a coughing child on the back is unhelpful and interferes with what is the most powerful expulsive force – the cough itself. If an aspirated foreign body is suspected, get the child calmly and quickly into the care of a competent anaesthetist for inhalational anaesthesia, direct laryngoscopic examination and removal of the obstructing object. If the situation is stable a portable X-ray may help locate radio-opaque objects.

Epiglottitis
Where epiglottitis is suspected the priorities are to minimise anxiety and fear and to proceed as rapidly as possible to inhalational anaesthesia, direct laryngoscopy and passing an endotracheal tube. Summon senior anaesthetic, paediatric and ENT assistance. Do not remove these children from the mother's arms. Venepuncture is contraindicated. X-ray examination may dangerously and unnecessarily delay definitive diagnosis and the X-ray department is a hazardous environment for the child with epiglottitis. Once the airway has been secured an intravenous line can be erected, blood cultures drawn and the concomitant septicaemia treatment commenced with appropriate antibiotics, e.g. ampicillin. Management for bacterial tracheitis is similar.

Laryngotracheobronchitis
The management of laryngotracheobronchitis will depend on the severity. Children with recession, stridor and laboured inspiration at rest should be admitted to hospital. Maintain hydration and observe for increasing airway obstruction. Administration of oxygen is rarely of value and may obscure signs of increasing distress. Administration of moist air in croupettes is of no clinical value and has the negative effects of frightening the child and obscuring the attending staff's view of the child. A single dose of dexamethasone or prednisolone probably helps. Nebulised saline and beta stimulants have no consistent effect. Nebulised raecemic adrenaline can be dramatically effective in diminishing laryngeal oedema but the effect is very shortlived. It has little place outside the intensive care unit. Usually when infants with laryngotracheobronchitis relax and sleep their stridor diminishes and the nursing effort will focus on relieving anxiety via parental reassurance. Where the child develops signs of increasingly severe narrowing, larngoscopy and intubation may be required. This occurs in less than 1 per cent of children admitted to hospital.

Key points

- Laryngomalacia causes mild stridor from birth, affected children thrive and recovery is spontaneous.
- The child with epiglottitis is toxic, drooling saliva, stridulous with minimal cough and is not hoarse.
- If epiglottitis is suspected – do not touch - get an anaesthetist urgently!
- The child with 'croup' has a barking cough, and is hoarse – steam is useless, steroids probably help.

Useful literature

- *Respiratory illness in children*, P. Phelan, L. Landau, and A. Olinsky (Blackwell, 1990).

PART II

Outpatient Presentations

19 Abnormal puberty

Puberty is the transitional period between the juvenile state and adulthood during which the adolescent growth spurt occurs with a change in body build and composition, the secondary sexual characteristics appear, fertility is achieved and profound psychological changes take place.

The stages of puberty have been described by Tanner and range from Stage 1 (no signs of puberty) to Stage 5 (full adult development). Testicular size is recorded as testicular volume using an orchidometer consisting of standard ovoids. The prepubertal testis is 2–3 ml in size and the adult varies between 12 and 25 ml. The first sign of puberty in a girl is usually breast development and in a boy, testicular enlargement.

Endocrinology of puberty

The mechanisms which trigger and modulate pubertal development are unknown. The initiation is partly genetically determined, and also influenced by environmental factors such as nutrition, chronic illness, stress and sport. Involved are the adrenal glands and the hypothalamo-pituitary-gonadal axis, with the hypothalamus releasing GnRH (gonadotrophin releasing hormone) stimulating the pituitary to release LH (luteinising hormone) and FSH (follicle stimulating hormone), which in turn stimulate the gonads to produce sex hormones.

The hypothalamo-pituitary-gonadal axis is very active during fetal life, in particular when sexual differentiation of the fetus takes place, and also at two months of age when a rise of sex steroids occurs. Following the second year of age, a quiescent period extends until 10 years of age during which time the hypothalamo-pituitary-gonadal axis is at rest. This is due to an inhibitory pathway which prevents activity; however, this pathway may be damaged by intracranial pathology which thus allows the stimulatory pathway to work unopposed and results in early puberty. After 10 years of age a reactivation of the hypothalamo-pituitary–gonadal axis occurs, resulting in raised plasma FSH and LH levels, leading to gonadal production of oestrogens or androgens and thus puberty starts. In girls the mean age of the first budding of the breast is 10.9 years (with a range of 8–13 years); menarche occurs at 13 years (with a range of 11–16 years). In boys the first growth of testis is observed at a mean age of 11.5 years (range 9–14 years); adult genitalia are observed from 14.5–18 years with a mean age of 15 years.

The individual variations at the time of onset of puberty are extremely wide and the time taken to pass through the various stages equally wide. The age of onset of puberty is approximately the same in both sexes. In girls puberty appears to be earlier than in boys and this is due to the fact that a girl's breast development is more evident to the casual observer than the increase in testicular size in boys. Also the adolescent height spurt in girls comes on average 2 years earlier than in boys. Approximately both sexes take 4 years from the beginning to the completion of puberty with a range between 2 and 5 years.

The age at which puberty occurs differs from population to population and changes with time. The age of menarche is influenced by numerous factors and has generally decreased during the past century in industrialised countries. Girls from higher socioeconomic classes and urban areas tend to mature earlier whilst those with poor nutrition, chronic illness, psychological problems or excessive exercise have a late menarche. Pubertal signs appearing in girls before the age of 8–9 years and in boys before 9–10 years are outside two standard deviations of the normal range and thus require investigation. Conversely girls and boys who show no signs of puberty by the age of 15 years should be investigated.

Precocious puberty

Precocious puberty can be defined as any signs of puberty occurring before the age of 8 years in a girl and 9 years in a boy. In girls early puberty is usually a benign condition, whereas in boys it is more often due to a pathological cause. Precocious puberty may be associated with full sexual development. The youngest mother in the literature is a Peruvian girl who delivered a 6 pound baby by caesarian section at the age of 5 years.

Causes of precocious puberty

1. Idiopathic precocious puberty is the most common type, especially in girls where it accounts for approximately 80 per cent. The cause is unknown and there is often a family history of early puberty.
2. Intracranial pathology including craniopharyngioma, hamartoma, glioma, tuberous sclerosis, neurofibromatosis or previous encephalitis, meningitis, or radiotherapy.
3. Hypothyroidism. The low plasma thyroxine level (T_4) stimulates the release of prolactin and gonadotrophins.
4. The McCune–Albright syndrome is the association of café-au-lait skin pigmentation and polyostotic fibrous dysplasia of bones with precocious puberty. This is a nonhereditary condition and occurs in both sexes.
5. Congenital adrenal hyperplasia is a condition where excessive androgens are produced by the adrenal cortex and may present in boys with signs of early pubertal development, including pubic hair, growth of the penis and increase in height. However, the adrenal androgens will not enlarge the testes. This condition in girls will cause virilising signs including pubic hair development, clitoromegaly, facial hair and increase in height. The adrenal androgens will not cause feminising signs such as breast development or menstruation.
6. Tumours producing ectopic gonadotrophins such as hepatoblastoma, adrenal cortical and testicular tumours producing androgens or ovarian cyst or tumour producing oestrogens.
7. Exogenous ingestion of sex hormones. This may occur from accidental ingestion of contraceptive pills or from the use of anabolic steroids as growth promoting agents.

Evaluation

History

Details of the nature and timing of the first signs and symptoms together with retrospective growth data should be obtained. It is important to establish whether the sequence of pubertal development is normal. An abnormal sequence is more likely to be pathological. Neurological symptoms such as headache, visual disturbances or ataxia should be sought and a past history which may have produced neurological damage. Obtain a family history, to include timing of puberty of parents, siblings and relatives. Enquiries should be made concerning any relatives dying suddenly or in infancy or having ambiguous genitalia which may suggest congenital adrenal hyperplasia. The possibility of accidental drug ingestion should be borne in mind.

Physical examination

Height and weight should be accurately recorded and the signs of puberty staged. Skin pigmentation suggestive of neurofibromatosis or the McCune–Albright syndrome should be looked for. The abdomen should be palpated for an adrenal, ovarian or hepatic tumour. Vaginal inspection for signs of oestrogenisation should be performed. A detailed neurological examination is essential.

Laboratory investigations

Plasma oestrogen levels will be elevated in a girl and plasma androgens in a boy with sexual precocity. A GnRH stimulation test will reveal high LH and FSH levels in central precocious puberty (this includes idiopathic and intracranial pathological causes) and suppressed levels will be found if the sex hormones are primarily derived from adrenal or gonadal pathology. Adrenal androgens are determined in a boy to exclude congenital adrenal hyperplasia. Thyroid function test should be done to exclude hypothyroidism and tumour markers such hCG and alpha fetoprotein levels may be indicated in boys.

Radiological assessment

Abdominal and pelvic ultrasonography may be used to detect an adrenal, hepatic, ovarian or testicular tumour. A CT or MRI brain scan is required in a child with central precocious puberty. A skeletal survey is performed if the McCune–Albright syndrome is suspected. The bone age is usually advanced.

Management

The primary condition is treated when possible, e.g. hypothyroidism, congenital adrenal hyperplasia and tumours. Where no treatable cause can be found therapy may be required to stop the rapid progression of secondary sexual development, the rapid increase in height and advance in bone age with ultimate short stature, and also to stop the psychological effects.

The two medications generally used are a GnRH agonist or cyproterone acetate:

- The GnRH agonist such as buserelin, leuprorelin, or triptorelin can be given by the intranasal route or as a monthly intramuscular depot preparation. It acts by inhibiting pituitary release of LH and FSH secretion by downregulating the receptors. The suppression of pubertal development is reversible within 3–12 months after discontinuation of therapy and clinical progression through puberty will resume normally. The GnRH agonist is effective in suppressing the sexual characteristics of puberty; however, as it has only been available for a relatively short time, it is not yet clear if it improves the final height which is usually compromised by precocious puberty.
- Cyproterone acetate in a daily dose of 70 mg/m^2 is taken orally in single or divided doses and suppresses pubertal signs by partially decreasing gonadotrophin release and gonadal steroidogenesis. It also has a suppressant effect on ACTH production and thus patients given cyproterone acetate should carry a steroid card and be warned of what action to take in an emergency. This medication will usually stop further pubertal development and psychosexual problems, but has little or no effect on the rapid increase in height and advance in bone age, which results in early closure of the epiphyses and a short final height.

  Psychological counselling and support is required for the child and family.

Premature thelarche

This is the occurrence of breast development in girls before the age of 5 years without the other physical changes of puberty. It is more common in early childhood. It is generally bilateral, but unilateral breast enlargement may occur. Usually the breasts remain the same size or regress slowly over several months. The explanation for premature thelarche is unclear. This may be due to an increased sensitivity of the breasts to prepubertal levels of circulating oestrogen or a small increased secretion or ingestion of oestrogen.

Extensive diagnostic evaluation of premature thelarche is not necessary; however, girls with early breast development must be examined at intervals of 3–6 months to monitor progression and to detect any other signs of precocious pubertal development such as rapid growth, development of pubic or axillary hair, or of menstruation. Any of these additional findings would indicate the need for further diagnostic investigation of complete precocious puberty.

Delayed puberty

The majority of children, particularly boys, with no signs of puberty by the age of 15 years have no organic disorder but represent the extreme end of the normal spectrum.

The differential diagnosis of delayed puberty includes:

1. constitutional growth delay which is the most common cause of delayed puberty. There is delay in the maturation of the hypothalamo-pituitary-gonadal axis and it is frequently familial.
2. endocrine causes of delayed puberty which may be divided into central, gonadal or peripheral groups.

- Central causes include gonadotrophin deficiency in isolation or combined with other evidence of hypothalamo-pituitary dysfunction, and can be detected by a GnRH test.
- Gonadal causes: this is the failure of the gonads to respond to stimulation by the gonadotrophins and occurs in chromosomal disorders such as Turner syndrome and Klinefelter's syndrome, and it also occurs with anorchia and may follow radiotherapy to the gonads. Gonadal failure is associated with raised levels of gonadotrophins. The physical features of Klinefelter's or Turner's syndromes may be present and the absent or very small testes will be found in anorchia. A human chorionic gonadotrophin (hCG) test will measure the ability of the testes to produce testosterone in response to LH. This is usually done by giving three intramuscular injections of hCG and measuring plasma testosterone prior to the first injection and on day 4. There will be a significant rise in plasma testosterone in the normal prepubertal boy.
- Peripheral causes include rare conditions such as defects of steroid biosynthesis and the androgen insensitivity syndrome which is associated with a female phenotype and a male chromosome karyotype.

3. Chronic illness, e.g. cystic fibrosis, severe asthma.

Investigations of delayed puberty

History and physical examination

A detailed history including family history and full physical examination is required to exclude a systemic illness, malnutrition, psychosocial stress and to obtain the previous growth rate of the child and the family timing of puberty. A complete neurological evaluation must be performed including assessment of the sense of smell (absent in Kallman's syndrome – anosmia and hypothalamic dysfunction).

Laboratory tests

Basal gonadotrophin levels will be elevated in primary gonadal failure. In patients with gonadotrophin deficiency the LH and FSH response to a GnRH test is significantly reduced. A serum prolactin level may be performed to exclude a rare prolactinoma. An hCG test will assess testicular ability to produce testosterone. Chromosome analysis is required to exclude Turner syndrome in a girl and Klinefelter's in a boy.

Radiological assessment

The bone age will be delayed. Pelvic ultrasonography is useful to assess ovarian and uterine maturation. A CT or MRI brain scan is indicated if a hypothalamo-pituitary tumour is suspected.

Treatment of delayed puberty

Constitutional delayed puberty often requires no treatment except height prediction and reassurance. Lack of pubertal development, however, associated with short stature due to the absence of the pubertal growth spurt may have marked psychological repercussions, particularly in boys. In such cases a short course of low dose oral oxandrolone is reasonable.

Key points

- Precocious puberty is idiopathic in 80 per cent of girls.
- The first sign of puberty is breast development in girls, testicular enlargement in boys.
- Precocious puberty leads to accelerated growth, early epiphyseal closure and a reduced adult height.
- Gonadotrophin releasing hormone agonists can suppress precocious puberty.
- 'Constitutional' delay is the most common cause of pubertal delay.
- Serious systemic illness, e.g. cystic fibrosis, often delays puberty.

Useful literature

- Normal puberty: physical characteristics and endocrinology, C. Brook and R. Stanhope. In: Clinical paediatric endocrinology, 2nd edition, C. Brook (ed.) (Blackwell, 1989)
- Physical growth, development and puberty – endocrinological aspects of puberty and adolescence, C. Kelnar. In: *Forfar and Arneil's textbook of paediatrics*, 4th edition, A. Campbell and N. McIntosh (eds) (Churchill Livingstone, 1992)
- Disorders of puberty, R. Stanhope and C. Brook. In: *Clinical paediatric endocrinology*, 2nd edition, C. Brook (ed.) (Blackwell, 1989)
- Physical growth, development and puberty – physical growth and puberty, J. Tanner. In: *Forfar and Arneil's textbook of paediatrics*, 4th edition, A. Campbell and N. McIntosh (eds) (Churchill Livingstone, 1992)
- The age of menarche in Irish girls, H. Hoey, J.M. Tanner, L.A. Cox (*Irish medical journal* 1986, 79, 283–286)

20 Asthma outpatient management

Introduction

Asthma affects 10–15 per cent of children. The diagnosis of asthma is clinical, and is usually straightforward. Management is predominantly at primary care level. Children with asthma will be seen in hospital clinics where there is a diagnostic problem or where control is unusually difficult. A particular problem is encountered with wheezy babies – is it asthma or self-limiting post-bronchiolitis wheeze? Time or therapeutic trials will help decide. The aim of management in childhood is to ensure a normal lifestyle, using the minimum amount of treatment. The natural history of childhood asthma is favourable. There are seasonal variations and a strong tendency towards spontaneous improvement with time so that we should always consider reducing medication when the condition is stable.

History

The key items in the history to indicate the adequacy of control are: school attendance, exercise tolerance, sleep disturbance and medication consumption. Ask if the child has missed school because of 'chest infection' or cough. School absence may be mistakenly attributed to chest infections, when clearly these have been episodes of asthma. Ask the child about participation in games –

parents tend to underestimated the frequency of exercise-induced asthma. Be alert to the fact that 'regular football' may mean standing around keeping goal! Ensure that the parents, or indeed the child, are not restricting activity to prevent symptoms. Nocturnal cough is common and may be the dominant symptom. Parents are more likely to complain, since children may not wake up with the cough.

Children with troublesome asthma should keep a record of the peak expiratory flow rate (PEFR). When assessing the diary card, be aware that your outpatient waiting rooms may be the site of feverish card filling!

Try to assess compliance with the current treatment regime. Ask the child to describe the daily medication routine. Check and record the doses given (you need to be familiar with capsule colours, etc.). Make sure the family know the difference between 'preventers' and 'relievers', and that they respond appropriately to increases in symptoms. A further useful assessment of compliance and severity is to ask how long it takes to 'use up' an inhaler. Excessive use of bronchodilator implies that prophylactic treatment is not adequate. Pay particular attention to side effects, especially where oral medications are used. Irritability, abdominal pain, vomiting, enuresis and

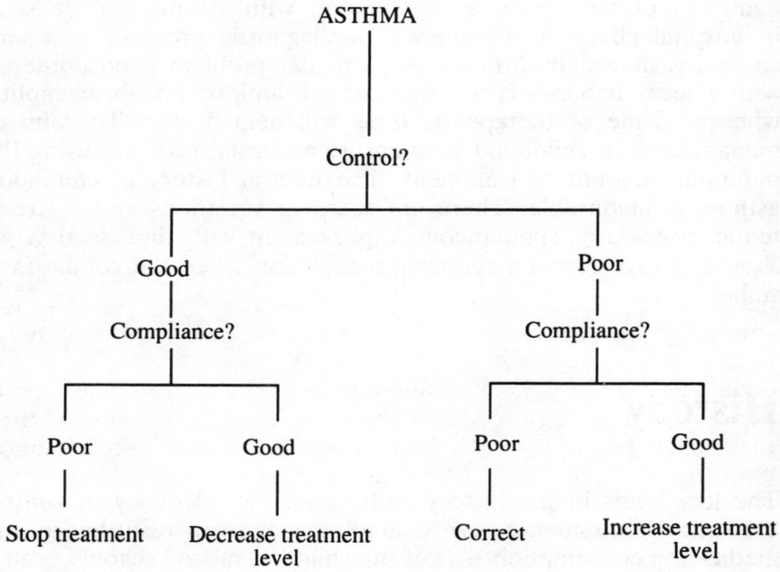

Fig. 20.1 Treatment decisions pathway in outpatient management of asthma

headache may all be caused by theophyllines. Enquire as to whether environmental precautions are being taken. Is there exposure to animal danders, passive smoking or excessive dust? Smoking, passive and active, is the most important environmental hazard – since it can be avoided.

Examination

Measurement of height and weight are important. There has been some concern that inhaled steroids, particularly in high doses, may interfere with linear growth. Conversely, poorly controlled asthma can also interfere with growth causing delayed puberty and poor weight gain. Inspect the chest for signs of hyperinflation and Harrison's sulci as these indicate poor control of asthma. Auscultation is frequently unrevealing, but the presence of rhonchi in a patient who denies symptoms suggests a problem with perception of dyspnoea. Measurement of the peak expiratory flow rate before and after bronchodilator is essential. Examine for evidence of allergic rhinitis and eczema. Ask the patient to demonstrate the inhaler technique.

Laboratory data

Investigations are generally unhelpful in routine management of asthma. Eosinophilia supports the diagnosis of asthma but will not influence treatment. Neutrophilia may be caused by stress (of an acute attack) or steroid therapy, not necessarily bacterial infection. Immunoglobin E levels are usually increased but have no prognostic or therapeutic implications.

Skin prick tests to common inhaled antigens may be requested by parents or referring physician. These are positive to some allergen in over 90 per cent of children with asthma – the most common antigens are house dust mite, grass pollen, animal danders and moulds. Interpretation is difficult, since 30 per cent of healthy controls have positive tests and skin tests do not always correlate with tests of bronchial provocation. Furthermore, dust mite reduction measures are of doubtful efficacy, grass pollen is difficult to avoid and pets are bad news anyway. (Cats have been defined as 'the crab grass on the lawn of civilisation'.) RAST tests provide similar, more expensive information on a blood sample.

Chest X-ray is occasionally of value to eliminate alternative pathologies and respiratory function tests may be of value particularly in severe cases where treatment is less effective than anticipated.

Treatment

The principles of treatment are:

1. Normal lifestyle using minimum of safest medication.
2. Inhaled treatment where possible because of increased efficacy and diminished side effects.
3. Single inhalation device for prophylaxis and symptom relief if possible.
4. Least frequent dosing to enhance compliance.
5. Regular reviews to assess the need for or the adequacy of treatment.

There are four broad levels of treatment depending on the severity of the asthma. Children with mild episodic asthma are given bronchodilators when symptomatic. Regular prophylactic treatment with sodium cromoglycate is offered when symptoms occur on most days or severe attacks occur more than once per month. If cromoglycate is inadequate after 6 weeks of trial with good compliance, then switch to inhaled steroids. Start with a dose of 200 μg twice daily, reducing if possible to the lowest dose compatible with good symptom control.

Sometime a higher dose of inhaled steroids is required. Theophyllines may be added, particularly if there are breakthrough symptoms at night (Table 20.1).

Regular alternate day oral steroids are rarely required. The role of long-acting bronchodilators in the management of childhood asthma is not clear as yet.

Table 20.1 Treatment levels

1. Beta-agonist as required
2. Sodium cromoglycate + 1
3. Inhaled steroid + 1
4. High dose inhaled steroids +/− theophylline + 1

Oral medication

The bronchodilators terbutaline, orciprenaline and salbutamol may all be given orally. In general, efficacy is reduced despite the relatively large dose and side effects, particularly tremor, are more common.

Theophyllines in syrup formulations are bitter tasting and require 6-hourly dosages. Therefore this drug is best given as a twice daily sustained release preparation. Children metabolise theophyllines more rapidly than adults and larger doses – approximately 20 mg per kg per day are necessary to achieve therapeutic blood levels. Eight-hourly dosage may be necessary in preschool children. It is best to start with a low dose, increasing gradually. This minimises side effects. Nevertheless, up to a third of children will discontinue treatment because of 'caffeine-like' toxicity - usually nausea, vomiting, irritability or insomnia. Blood or salivary levels may be valuable in monitoring. Because of the limitations of oral medications the inhaled route is preferable.

Inhaled medication

To be effective medication must be presented as particles of a size suitable for inhalation and deposition in the smaller airways. The choice of inhaler device rests between: nebuliser, dry powder devices, metered dose inhalers (MDI) with spacer or breath actuation. Unmodified MDI are generally useless in children under 10.

Nebulisers are driven by compressed air and generate a fine particle mist of medication which can be inhaled with little effort or co-operation. These are useful in very small children. Attention to detail is important. Ensure compressor output is adequate, i.e. approximately 8 litres per minute, and that it is regularly serviced. The nebuliser unit must be cleaned regularly and of a design that generates appropriate sized particles. Ensure that the optimal volume of drug solution is nebulised, 4 ml is usually appropriate. Inhalation through a mouthpiece is preferable. If a face mask is used, ensure that it is held snugly over the nose and mouth – if held away from the face, particles coalesce and efficacy is reduced.

Beta-agonist, cromoglycate and inhaled steroids can all be given by this method. Ensure the parents do not neglect regular prophylaxis; the nebulisation times of 10–20 minutes at least twice daily tend to reduce compliance. Give the parents a treatment plan so that they realise when to seek help, for example if there is a poor response to nebulised beta-agonist or the child is so breathless that he is unable to talk. In older children, nebulisers have no advantage over MDI plus spacer for delivery of beta-agonist, if equivalent doses are used.

Dry powder devices include the spinhaler, rotahaler, dischaler and turbohaler. The characteristics vary, as does the inspiratory flow necessary for optimal drug delivery. Children as young as 3 years can use these devices. They are portable and discreet – this is particularly important to schoolgoing children. In very severe dyspnoea, however, the child may be unable to generate adequate inspiratory flow to activate the device.

Metered dose inhalers deliver, at great velocity, a suspension of drug with a volatile agent – usually freon. The freon evaporates rapidly leaving a cloud of small particles. Children under 10 are rarely able to co-ordinate actuation of the canister with inhalation so that much of the drug impacts on the oropharynx and lung deposition is suboptimal. Spacing chambers such as the volumatic, nebuhaler, fisonair and aerochamber have been developed to overcome these co-ordination problems. The drug 'cloud' is held in the spacer and can then be inhaled via the one-way valve – the timing and mode of breathing is not critical. The 'autohaler' is a device that links initiation of inhalation and actuation of the MDI and studies of its use in children suggest that it is valuable. Freon is a chloroflurocarbon (CFC) and will probably be withdrawn because of depletion of the ozone layer. Alternative delivery agents are being assessed.

Cost is a further consideration. MDIs are generally cheapest – spacers are an additional 'once off' cost. Dry powder devices are more expensive. Nebuliser/compressor units are expensive and the drug solutions for these devices are particularly costly.

Decisions

Decisions are based on the answers to two questions. Is asthma controlled adequately? Is treatment being delivered effectively – i.e. is there good compliance, proper technique and adequate dosage? (Fig. 20.1).

Table 20.2 Devices

	Advantages	**Disadvantages**
Nebuliser	No co-operation	Cost/time
Dry powder	Convenience	Cost, acute attacks, co-operation required
MDI plus spacer	Effective most ages, all times	Bulky devices, ozone depletion

Where symptom control is adequate and has been for several months it is reasonable to reduce to the next lowest level of treatment. Conversely where symptom control is poor despite adequate compliance with the prescribed treatment, then an increase in level of treatment is appropriate.

Behaviour modification may be necessary if there are indications of poor compliance or adverse environmental factors. The choice of inhaler method may need to be reviewed if there are shortcomings in technique. In general the basic decision concerns the level of treatment. The 'four step' management levels are indicated in Table 20.1.

Many children with asthma, particularly those with episodic asthma, will outgrow their symptoms. Children with persistent asthma, particularly if this is severe and accompanied by other atopic illnesses, will tend to have symptoms to adulthood though these may diminish in severity in adolescence. Patient education in asthma is a continuous process. The provision of written material is helpful and a willingness to answer questions is essential.

Key points

- School attendance, exercise tolerance, sleep disturbance and bronchodilator consumption are key indicators of asthma control.
- Avoid passive smoking.
- Children with severe asthma should monitor peak flow rate twice daily.
- Always check inhaler technique.
- Keep treatment regimes simple.
- If control is good, consider reducing treatment.

Useful literature

- *Respiratory illness in children*, P. Phelan, L. Landau and A. Olinsky (Blackwell, 1990)

21 Behavioural problems

As part of effective child rearing, parents need to train their children to develop appropriate behaviour patterns to enable them to live happily and effectively in the real world. This process is discipline. Discipline should foster creativity and spontaneity, whilst encouraging orderliness, self-control and obedience. The word discipline now has a rather negative, punitive image, but for it to be effective it must be gently and lovingly applied.

Children naturally want their parents' attention, love and praise. Where behaviour is rewarded it will persist. If behaviour is ignored it will not be repeated. Most behaviour problems can be reduced to the child performing the behaviour that is unwittingly being rewarded by the parents. Even where parents react angrily or negatively to a behaviour pattern, this may be mistakenly interpreted by the child as reward, since it may be the only time they get their parents' exclusive attention. Any form of behaviour that will produce the desired response will be repeated and very frequently the child does not have a problem – the parent does!

Smacking has no place in discipline. It teaches children that they will be able to impose their will by physical force on smaller people. They also find it difficult to understand how somebody who professes to love them can hit them. Smacking may ease the parents' tension transiently but is likely to result in a surge of guilt with a very confusing message for the child who is smacked and shortly afterwards comforted.

Where some form of 'punishment' is deemed necessary the 'time out' is probably the most effective. This consists of an absence of physical, verbal or visual communications for a period of time. To be effective it must be instituted soon after the undesired behaviour, the child must know the reason for the time out and it should end when the child is quiet. In isolation this method is ineffective so that it must be coupled with positive reinforcement for appropriate behaviour.

Behaviour problems occur from time to time in all families. Their spectrum ranges from transient loss of control, which is normal, to complete loss of control by either parent or child. The commonest behaviour problems involve eating, sleeping, bowel and bladder control, crying, destructive behaviour, hyperactivity and temper tantrums. Crying and constipation are dealt with elsewhere. This section will deal briefly with the remaining problems.

Eating

Parents commonly complain that their child 'will not eat anything'. Children are usually in the toddler age group and the problem tends to begin between 12 and 18 months. At this time the infant's growth velocity slows dramatically and caloric requirements also decline. It may therefore be perplexing for parents to find that their 2-year-old eats much less than a 6-month-old baby. This may understandably cause some anxiety and parents will then try to encourage the toddler to eat more at meal times. This can then become an elaborate game. From the child's point of view this is wonderful! He is the centre of attention, fiddling delicately with his dinner or alternatively engaging in enjoyable games as make-believe 'helicopters' of food are ferried to his mouth by his approving parents.

The main point in clinical evaluation is to monitor the child's height, weight and nutrition. This is invariably normal though it can be difficult to convince the parents that normal growth is possible in a child who apparently ingests no calories! On closer questioning it usually transpires that the child is having small frequent snacks or drinking large quantities of milk, so that he has no additional requirement for calories at meal times. Simple reassurance, elimination of snacks between meals and meal presentation on a 'take it or leave it' basis will resolve the problem.

In later childhood refusal to eat may be due to anorexia nervosa which is associated with significant weight loss and additional psychological problems. The child, usually female, may try to disguise the poor eating by binging with subsequent vomiting. Where organic causes of anorexia are excluded, referral to child psychiatry services is indicated.

Sleeping problems

The normal pattern of sleep varies from child to child and from time to time. It depends on the child's health, presence or absence of stress affecting the child or parents, the personality of the child and the parents, and the tolerance of the parents at any given time. Irregular sleep disturbances occur in up to 20 per cent of 2-year-olds and between 10 per cent and 15 per cent of children aged 3–4. The common ongoing sleep disorders which result in parents seeking help are:

1. persistent difficulty in settling at bed-time,
2. excessive wakening, and
3. night terrors and nightmares.

In evaluating this problem again be aware that the parent is the one with the problem. The child is usually quite happy with the situation, it is the parents who are exhausted from poor sleep. Inappropriate 'rewarding' is extremely common in this situation. From the child's point of view parental attention at night time is likely to be high grade – there is no television, no meals to prepare, no other children or neighbours to entertain. It is easy to see how the child may interpret this attention as 'reward'.

Difficulty in settling

This problem generally occurs in toddlers. There may be a precipitating emotional upset, for instance hospitalisation or death of a relative. More common reasons are lack of a bedtime routine designed to help the child wind down, overstimulation at bedtime by vigorous games or exciting television, or fear of the dark. It can also be an attention seeking device. Younger children find it a lot more interesting to be with their parents at bedtime and may cry when they leave them. This behaviour will be reinforced if parents give the child a bottle or lift the child. If crying persists parents may end up lying with the child or bringing the child into their own bed. On occasions difficulty in settling occurs in children who are 'overtired', irritable and overstimulated as a result of parental attempts to quieten them. Settling problems in older children and adolescents may result from anxiety over mundane matters such as acne or interpersonal relations. Disturbance of the sleep–wake cycle may also result from late bedtime and late rising or consumption of coffee or alcohol prior to bedtime. Difficulty getting to sleep may be a symptom of anxiety/depression; early morning waking may be an indication of endogenous depression.

Management depends on the likely precipitating factors. It is vital that the parents are given an insight into the child's view of events. An appropriate bedtime should be chosen and a routine designed to gradually wind the child down should be evolved. For example, after the child's bath he goes to bed, is read a story and the light is turned out. The room should not be bright, and parents should calmly withdraw. Bedtime drinks should be avoided as they are bad for teeth and may reinforce the unwanted behaviour pattern. Parents should agree on a bedtime routine and also on their response to the inevitable attempts of the child to restore the previous pattern.

Excess waking

Some 10–20 per cent of children under three continue to wake during the night. On rare occasions this may be due to a physical problem such as pruritus due to eczema or threadworms, a wet bed from enuresis or upper airway obstruction from adenoidal enlargement. More commonly excess waking is due to a failure to develop a normal rhythm of sleep. Many reasons contribute to this failure including the child's temperament – (low adaptability, low sensory threshold) and parental responses. If the child is settled in different places each night, the unfamiliar surroundings when he wakens may cause anxiety. If the child is given a bottle each time he wakes, sleeping through the night takes much longer to establish. If the parents bring the child into their bed this will actively encourage waking.

Physical causes clearly need to be identified. The normal sleep stages and patterns should be explained to parents and parental anxieties need to be addressed. Manipulating the child into a more 'adult-oriented' sleep pattern involves stopping the unwitting rewarding of night-time waking. This is easier said than done! Parents need to agree on a plan, either a phased scheme or an abrupt change. The essence of the behaviour change is that the child's waking must not be rewarded and that adequate night-time sleeping should be praised.

Night terrors

These occur early in sleep, during the non-rapid eye movement phase of sleep. Their severity ranges from mild confusion to incoherent babbling to the screaming of an apparently terrified child. The child remains asleep, so communication is not possible. The episodes generally end within five minutes and the child has no memory of them. Nightmares are frightening dreams which occur during rapid eye movement sleep. The child may wake up terrified by the dream. Precipitating causes such as TV programmes, stories or recent trauma are usually identifiable. When the child has woken up the parents should provide comfort and reassurance.

Temper tantrums

These are one of the common ways in which assertive toddlers try to gain control of the environment. They typically occur between 18 months and 3 years, a stage where the child is learning that he cannot have what he wants instantly, but where he has not yet developed the concept of 'later'. Tantrums are more common where the child is tired, hungry or frustrated. The child may hit or kick his parents or lie on the floor kicking, screaming or head banging. The parents are frequently concerned that the child may do himself an injury and as a result will accede to the demand and subsequently may try to avoid conflict. Alternatively the parents may smack the child. One way or the other, the unacceptable behaviour becomes reinforced. Temper tantrums occur in virtually all children and where persistent, advising the parents to ignore them and not to give in to them is effective.

Breathholding attacks are a more sophisticated form of temper tantrum. Precipitating events may include frustration or minor injury. The child may cry for 10–15 seconds before holding his breath, becoming cyanosed, hypotonic and unconscious. When the child becomes unconscious, breathing spontaneously starts again and there is rapid recovery though there may be pallor for some time afterwards. On occasions there may even be some clonic jerking. The management is the same as for temper tantrums though parents require firm reassurance, as these events are often terrifying and from the child's point of view, may be extremely effective.

Destructive or antisocial behaviour

A child who has no regard for norms of behaviour or the needs of others is 'spoilt'. Boundaries to acceptable behaviour have not been defined by the care givers and the natural curiosity of the child will lead him on to try new and exciting behaviours. Paradoxically this 'boundary free' existence may cause ongoing anxiety for the child, lacking the security of knowing what is and what is not acceptable.

Parents may complain bitterly that they 'can never take our eyes off him' or that the child is 'impossible'. Punitive methods will usually have been employed to no avail. Sometimes parents will relate that they spend most of the day shouting at the child – the full-blown 'spoilt brat' scenario. The key observation is that the child is merely producing what he sees as the behaviour his parents want. Parental verbal abuse may be perceived by the child as high quality parental attention and he is merely trying to please! It may be very difficult to convince the parents that the child is responding normally to abnormal cues. Simple advice may suffice, but in resistant cases referral to child guidance services will help. Parents are likely to shop around alternative practitioners in the belief that the behaviour is due to some form of food allergy or poisoning from food preservatives. Much of the apparent positive response produced by dietary manipulation is through the concomitant change in the parents' attitudes – whereby they expect good behaviour and are likely to praise it when it occurs.

Hyperactivity

Attention deficit disorder is one of the lasting transatlantic paradoxes. This syndrome of short attention span, perpetual movement, inability to complete tasks and impulsiveness is said to be present in 3 per cent of the population. The condition is commonly diagnosed in North America and usually treated with amphetamines. Such diagnosis and treatment are exceedingly rare in the British Isles. All paediatricians will be familiar with hyperactive and destructive behaviour in handicapped children. This commonly improves with age and also with behaviour modification. Parents sometimes complain that their children are 'hyper'. This is usually a misinterpretation of normal surges of activity at particular times of the day. Alternative practitioners will often diagnose food allergy or ascribe symptoms to ingestion of preservatives or caffeine. By and large 'physical' explanations for hyperactivity are in the realm of fiction. Management is along the behavioural lines emphasised earlier – rewarding task completion, spending time with the child to develop interest in activities and providing a structure for the child's play.

Key points

- If a behaviour is ignored long enough, it stops.
- If behaviour is rewarded, it persists.
- If a child is growing normally, caloric intake is adequate.
- Children will always get enough sleep.
- Children can not sustain significant injury in tantrums, or breathholding.
- Hyperactivity is not caused by diet.

Useful literature

- *The normal child*, R. Illingworth (Churchill Livingstone, 1991)

22 Chronic diarrhoea

Introduction

Diarrhoea persisting for more than 2 weeks is defined as chronic. This presentation accounts for many outpatient consultations. In most cases the aetiology is benign and clinical evaluation with basic investigations can determine cause.

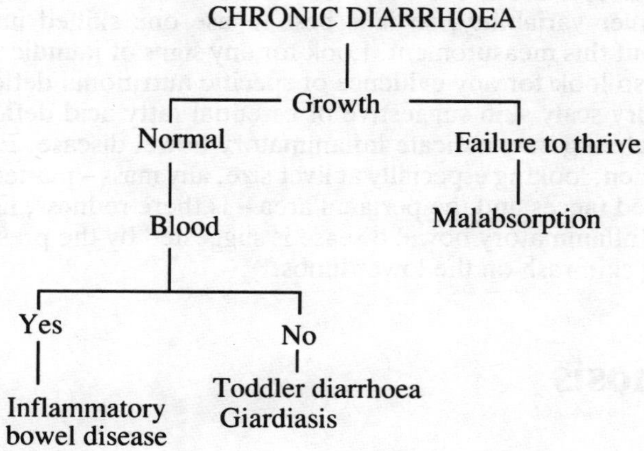

Fig. 22.1 Diagnostic pathway for the child with chronic diarrhoea

History

Define the duration of symptoms, frequency of stools per day, stool consistency and get some indication of stool volume. Ask if there are any precipitating, aggravating or relieving factors. Is there any perianal excoriation, pain or alternating constipation? The presence of blood or recognisable foods in the stool should be specifically elicited. Enquire as to the child's general well-being, appetite and energy level. In the past history, pay particular attention to neonatal bowel habits, feeding practice in infancy and previous surgery. Socio-economic factors, especially overcrowding, poor sanitation, poverty and malnutrition, would be very relevant. Worldwide, these factors account for most morbidity. The family history may be positive in coeliac disease or inflammatory bowel disease.

Examination

Measurement of height and weight is the most important investigation. Additional nutritional information would be obtained by assessment of skinfold thicknesses and mid arm circumference. Skinfold thickness is measured with a callipers over the triceps and subscapular area and gives a useful measure of subcutaneous fat. There is large interobserver variability, so it is best to use one skilled nurse for carrying out this measurement. Look for any signs of jaundice or pallor and also look for any evidence of specific nutritional deficiencies (such as dry scaly skin suggestive of essential fatty acid deficiency). Digital clubbing may indicate inflammatory bowel disease. Examine the abdomen, looking especially at liver size, any mass – matted bowel or impacted faeces and the perianal area – is there redness, fistula or fissures? Inflammatory bowel disease is suggested by the presence of ulcerating skin rash on the lower limbs.

Diagnosis

When spurious diarrhoea due to chronic constipation is excluded there are three main diagnostic categories to be considered:

1. normal growth and examination,
2. poor growth,
3. bloody diarrhoea.

Normal growth

Toddler diarrhoea

This is the commonest cause seen in outpatient clinics. Affected children are well with normal appetite and growth. The diarrhoea is often episodic and stools characteristically contain recognisable foodstuff, typically vegetables. It is also referred to as 'peas and carrots diarrhoea'. The condition is self-limiting, usually clearing before the third birthday. An increase in bowel transit time, mediated by prostaglandins, is thought to be responsible. Treatment is generally not necessary, though loperamide may be used for symptomatic relief in severe cases.

Transient lactase deficiency

This may follow severe gastroenteritis, the mucosal injury resulting in loss of brush border enzyme. Since the stool will contain excess lactose, it is acidic and causes perianal irritation. Diagnosis rests on demonstrating reducing sugars in the stool. Treatment is by exclusion of lactose from the diet for 1 or 2 weeks.

Giardiasis

Infection with *Giardia lamblia* may cause protracted diarrhoea with or without malabsorption. Stool examination may need to be repeatedly performed to make the diagnosis. Treatment is with metronidazole.

Poor growth

Cystic fibrosis

Though rare, this condition presents with malabsorption in almost half the cases. Diarrhoea is typically present from birth and the stools are greasy with a penetrating odour. Perianal excoriation, rectal prolapse and accompanying chest symptoms all suggest the diagnosis. Analysis of sweat electrolyte levels is the definitive test. This may be technically difficult in infants and measurement of immunoreactive trypsin in blood is a useful test in the first 6 weeks of life. Genotyping may be helpful in diagnosis of borderline cases. Management is a multidisciplinary effort involving chest physiotherapy, nutritional support, vigorous treatment of respiratory infections and regular clinical reviews.

Coeliac disease

Caused by a permanent intolerance to gluten in the diet, this condition has protean manifestations. Symptoms are rare in early infancy, unless wheat containing foods have been introduced. Diarrhoea is common, stools are bulky, greasy and offensive. Additional features include anorexia, vomiting, abdominal distension, muscle wasting and general misery! Though the incidence of the disease is declining and cases tend to present in later childhood, this is an important, treatable cause of chronic diarrhoea. Diagnosis is based on demonstrating villous atrophy in a jejunal biopsy, a clinical and histological response to a gluten free diet and relapse on re-exposure. Measurement of antigliaden antibodies (IgA) may be helpful in diagnosis and assessing response to treatment. A gluten free diet must be continued indefinitely because of the increased risk of intestinal lymphoma in later life.

Sugar intolerance

Permanent intolerance of lactose, sucrose or maltose will lead to osmotic diarrhoea when the offending sugar is ingested. Diagnosis is based on the suggestive history and the demonstration of the relevant sugars in the stool. Treatment is by exclusion.

Rare conditions

Schwachmann syndrome consists of exocrine pancreatic insufficiency and cyclical neutropenia. Bacterial overgrowth in blind loops of bowel, possibly as a result of surgery, necrotising enterocolitis or Crohn's disease, may present with malabsorption. Short-gut syndrome follows extensive resection, especially procedures involving resection of the ileocaecal valve. Deficiency of IgA, acquired immune deficiency and agammaglobulinaemia can all cause chronic diarrhoea. Abetalipoproteinaemia and hypoparathyroidism can also cause steatorrhoea.

Some children with chronic diarrhoea defy precise categorisation. These are often infants who have had complicated medical and surgical problems and appear to be intolerant of all forms of dietary nutrients. A period of parenteral nutrition is often necessary.

Bloody diarrhoea

Ulcerative colitis

In infancy, this condition is frequently a manifestation of cow's milk protein intolerance. Diarrhoea is profuse, watery and bloody. Toxic dilatation of the colon is potentially lethal. Diagnosis is by endoscopy and biopsy. Exclusion diet is usually curative in infants.

Crohn's disease

This is usually a disorder of adolescence. Symptoms may be vague and delayed diagnosis is frequent. Weight loss is common. Diagnosis is by endoscopy, barium studies or a combination. Management remains controversial – elemental diet, surgery, antibiotics and immunosuppressives all have some role.

Investigations

The necessity for and choice of investigations will depend on the clinical evaluation. Where the situation is unclear some basic tests will provide reassurance or point to the need for a more detailed assessment. Much information can be gleaned from a blood count, biochemistry profile and stool examination.

Haematology

Measurement of haemoglobin and red cell indices will give an indication of whether there is any deficiency of iron, folic acid or B12. Iron deficiency is commonly nutritional but may be associated with malabsorption. Folic acid deficiency will cause a macrocytosis and is suggestive of coeliac disease. B12 deficiency may be due to absence of terminal ileum following neonatal surgery. Elevated white cell count and platelet count suggest an ongoing inflammatory process. The erythrocyte sedimentation rate is invariably elevated in active inflammatory bowel disease. Examination of the blood film may give clues as to particular conditions, e.g. characteristic appearances of acanthocytosis in children with a betalipoproteinaemia.

Biochemistry

Disturbance of electrolyte levels may suggest the need for intravenous treatment and can also be helpful in defining aetiology. For instance the rare chloride losing enteropathy will cause profound hypochloraemia. Elevated levels of alkaline phosphatase may be due to liver dysfunction or bone disease caused by rickets. Inflammatory bowel disease may cause an associated cholangitis. Hypoalbuminaemia suggests either malnutrition or chronic liver disease. Hypocalcaemia can simply be associated with hypoalbuminaemia or may point to an underlying hypoparathyroidism-associated steatorrhoea.

Stool bacteriology

Examination of the stool for ova parasites and pathogenic bacteria should be part of routine evaluation. These organisms tend to cause shortlived diarrhoea, though cryptosporidium may cause chronic symptoms.

Stool biochemistry

Examination of liquid stool to measure pH and to check for the presence of sugar and fat is important. Collection of specimens may be a problem, with the liquid stool soaking into the absorbent napkin. Reversing the napkin for a period of time may allow efficient collection of specimens.

Key points

- Spurious diarrhoea may be due to chronic constipation with overflow incontinence.
- Toddler diarrhoea is the most common cause.
- Measurement of growth and nutrition is the key observation.
- Coeliac disease is now rare.
- Infantile colitis is usually allergic.

Useful literature

- *Harries paediatric gastroenterology*, P. Milla and D. Muller (Churchill Livingstone, 1988)

23 Constipation

Introduction

Constipation is a common problem in the paediatric age group. It warrants careful consideration since there may be a serious underlying problem. The prognosis is in general good, even in the severe cases which can progress to a stage of fecal retention with overflow incontinence.

Constipation may be caused by any factor which interferes with the normal sequence of defecation, considered below:

1. Colonic propulsion: the descending and sigmoid colon are the fecal storage organs which will, at intervals, propel the feces into the rectum.
2. Rectal sensation: The rectum has a sensing mechanism which

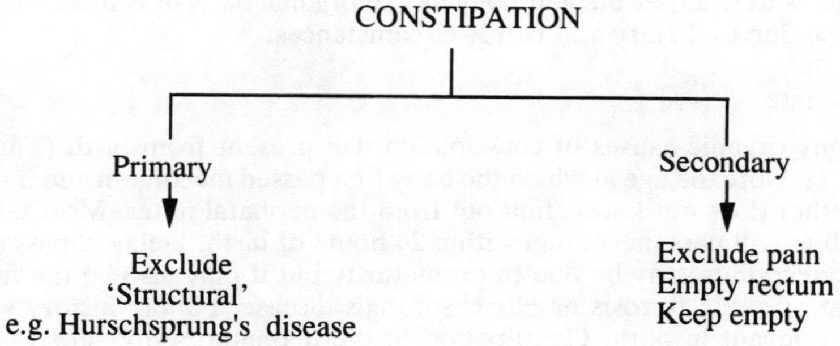

Fig. 23.1 Management pathway for constipation

relays at S2–4. The stretch receptors respond to the arrival of feces, eliciting rectal contraction.

3. Relaxation of the internal sphincter, which is mediated through Meissner's and Auerbach's plexuses.
4. The next mechanism is under voluntary control and may be either:

- defecation which can progress with the aid of a Valsalva manoeuvre;
- activation of the continence mechanism: there is voluntary contraction of the external sphincter and the puborectalis sling part of the levator ani muscle. Defecation is postponed and the internal sphincter regains its normal tone.

Any obstruction in the area of the rectum, internal sphincter or anus can interfere with the normal process of defecation.

History

Constipation usually presents during infancy or in the toddler age group. It is important at the outset to establish whether the report is valid. Many young babies go through very impressive Valsalva manoeuvres while defecating, but the frequency and type of stool are normal and there is no underlying problem. If the pattern of defecation is normal and straining is the only cause of anxiety, there is no indication for treatment or investigation. Stool frequency is related to feeding volume especially in the first 6 months of life.

Perhaps the most important point in the history is to establish the age of onset of the constipation. The age of onset may also be a major clue as to whether the aetiology has an organic basis or is more likely to be due to dietary and family circumstances.

Neonate

Many organic causes of constipation will present from birth (Table 23.1). Note the age at which the baby first passed meconium and if the mother does not know, find out from the neonatal notes. Most term babies will pass meconium within 24 hours of birth. Delayed passage of meconium may be due to prematurity but it may also be the first sign of cystic fibrosis or Hirschsprung's disease. Family history will be relevant in both. Constipation in the neonatal period should be regarded as organic in the first place. Obstructive constipation may be caused by a meconium plug, a presacral teratoma, anorectal malformations or an ectopic anus. Hirschsprung's disease is due to failure of relaxation of the internal sphincter as a result of failed migration of neuroblasts to the distal bowel between the sixth and twelfth week of gestation. Apart from classic Hirschsprung's disease, which will present as gut obstruction, it is important also to recognise ultra short segment Hirschsprung's disease. Constipation is a feature of the prune belly syndrome and neuromuscular disorders, especially spina bifida. The aetiology may be similar in sacral agenesis but the diagnosis will not be obvious until an X-ray is taken.

Infancy

Constipation is more likely to be 'functional' beyond the neonatal period. Clayden has usefully separated the stages of the common functional types of constipation into:

1. dietary
2. reluctance
3. retention
4. acquired megarectum stage.

These stages tend to affect different age groups.

The main dietary problem in late infancy is due to prolonged bottle feeding, which is the commonest cause of a low residue diet in this age group. Because the calorie intake from milk is adequate, the babies have no interest in a wider diet at weaning time. Their parents perceive the problem as anorexia, selective for normal nutritious

Table 23.1 Organic causes of constipation

Neonate	Meconium ileus Meconium plug Hirschsprung's disease Pseudo Hirschsprung's Ultra short segment disease Presacral teratoma Ectopic anus Anorectal malformations Sacral agenesis Hypothyroidism
Infancy	Coeliac disease Infantile hypercalcaemia Nephrogenic diabetes insipidus Renal tubular acidosis

foods. These babies are thriving because their calorie intake from milk easily meets the needs for growth and weight gain and it often passes unrecognised that the important malnutrition is iron deficiency. Iron deficiency is probably an important cause of this selective anorexia. This diet provides very little fecal residue and as a result, the stools tend to be hard and may cause an anal fissure. Reduced fluid intake, vomiting or polyuria may aggravate the tendency towards hard stools. During infancy, constipation may be an unusual presentation of coeliac disease.

Toddler

In this age group some children tend to withhold because of painful defecation. Withholding may also occur in toddlers who are determined to frustrate their parent's potty training regimens. This group may go on to a stage of fecal retention and this is especially true in those babies with a large rectal capacity.

Megarectum may develop as the rectum gradually becomes desensitised. Normal children will be continent by the age of 3, but it may be difficult to distinguish the late acquisition of continence from the onset of retention with overflow incontinence.

School age

The final stage of retention with overflow incontinence is commonest in the school age group. This may give rise to 'spurious' diarrhoea. Constipation may begin at this age, when withholding may occur because of simple circumstances such as poor school toilet facilities.

The term encopresis is sometimes used to describe soiling as a result of retention with overflow incontinence. The term should more correctly be reserved for non-retentive soiling. The latter problem is rare and is in the domain of child psychiatry. In the school age group, constipation may also present as recurrent abdominal pain. School children with cystic fibrosis may develop with meconium ileus equivalent. Constipation is also a very common problem in children with mental handicap and especially those who have an associated immobility due to physical handicap. Finally, constipation may result from a combination of minor factors such as diet, immobilisation from acute illness and stress.

Examination

The general approach to clinical examination should be like that of any other paediatric condition with establishment of the centiles for height and weight to ensure that the child is thriving and thus making any underlying systemic disorder unlikely. The nervous system should be examined with particular reference to the lower limbs and the tendon reflexes of the knees and ankle joints. Spinal cord problems such as diastematomyelia may present with a limp or bladder problems, but constipation may also be a feature. The abdomen should be palpated to detect fecal masses.

The anus should be inspected carefully. This is most easily done in babies and toddlers if the mother or carer holds the baby in the lithotomy position facing the examiner. A baby or toddler may be made very comfortable in this position and an excellent view of the perineum can be easily obtained without distress. The anus should be

Table 23.2 The evaluation of constipation

		True	*False*
Onset	Neonate:	Organic disease (Table 23.1)	Normal Variation
	Infancy:		Low residue diet
		Reduced fluids	Straining
	Toddler:	Withholding + fissure	
	School age:	Retention + overflow	
Examination	Growth and weight gain		
	Abdomen:	Faeces/pelvic mass	
	Anus:	Location	
		Trauma	
		Patulous	
	Rectum:	Sphincter tone	
		Faeces/mass	
		Gush sign	
	CNS:	S2–4	
Investigate	Plain film of abdomen		
	Rectal biopsy		
	Barium enema		
	Anal manometry		
	Haematology/biochemistry		
Management	Paediatric surgery		
	Diet		
	Laxatives		
	Enemas – antegrade continence		
	Child psychiatry		

inspected for fissures which tend to occur at six and twelve o'clock and there may be associated anal tags in that position. The anal position should be noted and this should be midway between the fornix and the tip of the coccyx. Anterior displacement of the anus can cause problems, especially in females, and is probably underdiagnosed.

In neurological disorders, the anus may be patulous. The integrity of the somatic nervous system can be tested by stimulating the rectal mucosa with a cotton wool bud and this should result in an anal wink. Skin sensation from the perianal region to the sitting area will test the S2–4 dermatomes. The anal region also needs to be inspected for evidence of trauma. Sometimes children with constipation and overflow incontinence are subjected to repeated treatments with suppositories and enemas at home resulting in excoriation of the perianal region. The question of sexual abuse needs to be kept in mind. The problems of differentiating reflex anal dilatation caused by sexual abuse or constipation are now well known. Reflex anal dilatation is not pathognomonic of child sexual abuse.

Rectal examination should then be conducted with the baby still in the lithotomy position. On occasion rectal examination may cause such distress that it is best deferred, unless crucial diagnostic information is anticipated. Rectal tone can be assessed to some extent with the finger. In the newborn it is often possible to get above the obstruction in Hirschsprung's disease and this will result in the so-called 'gush' sign. There is a sudden whoosh of liquid meconium and gas as the distended gut deflates. The sphincter tone may be tight in ultra short segment Hirschsprung's disease and there will be no feces in the rectum in Hirschsprung's disease. Rectal examination may relieve the obstruction caused by a meconium plug in the newborn. In the commoner types of constipation, starting with the dietary stage and going through to the reluctant, retaining and megarectum stages, there is likely to be feces in the rectum. The sphincter tone is likely to be fairly lax in the various stages unless the external sphincter is being actively contracted because of local pain. In infancy, presacral teratoma may cause constipation and is palpable on digital examination of the rectum. It is important to diagnose this condition early; though the teratoma is benign in infancy, it later undergoes malignant change.

Investigations

A plain film of abdomen together with a full blood count are the only investigations usually required in the common types of constipation. The plain film of abdomen will show the extent of constipation and this simple investigation has been shown to correlate well with other measures of transit time using radio-opaque markers. A full blood count is necessary to detect the commonly associated iron deficiency anaemia, which is nearly always of dietary origin.

If Hirschsprung's disease is suspected, then a rectal biopsy is necessary. This procedure should only be undertaken by an expert, otherwise unsatisfactory samples will necessitate repetition of the investigation. In the past, barium enemas were frequently used to exclude Hirschsprung's disease. In practice, a barium enema should only be required to confirm the extent of this disorder. Anorectal manometry is useful, but is only available in specialised centres. Other investigations are necessary when an unusual underlying disorder is suspected.

Management

Emphasis should be placed on early evaluation to exclude disease in the cases which present during the neonatal period or early infancy. The common type of functional constipation may respond to simple dietary advice but the management becomes more difficult as the problem becomes long-standing and progressive. In the rare cases when constipation is due to organic disease, then clearly the management is principally that of the underlying disorder.

In the more common type of non-organic constipation, the problem should be dealt with using oral medication. Often, these children are subjected to treatment using suppositories and enemas, resulting in only temporary relief and causing discomfort and fear. Simple laxative treatment using lactulose or liquid paraffin will often give the required result. If these simple laxatives are inadequate then it may be necessary to add a stimulant preparation such as senna or bisacodyl.

In long-standing cases, where there is retention and overflow incontinence, hospital admission may be required. In these cases, very large doses of laxatives can be given by mouth rather than using enemas. The result is more often the first step towards a permanent cure rather than the temporary remission provided by enemata.

It is better to defer high residue diet and bulk laxatives in severe cases with long-standing fecal retention until the backlog of feces has been cleared. The duration of laxative therapy is very difficult to determine and parents need to be advised that they should withdraw therapy very slowly and be prepared to revert to higher doses if there is a tendency to relapse. It is important to advise the parents that there is no correct dose of these laxatives and the treatment needs to be individually prescribed for each child.

Children who are soiling will very often have had an extremely rough time at school and advice from child psychiatrists may help. Child psychiatry support is mandatory in those children who have non-retentive soiling.

Children who are mentally handicapped often have intractable constipation which is very resistant to therapy. The antegrade continence enema has recently been described and this may prove to be a useful method in those particularly difficult cases associated with physical and mental handicap.

Key points

- Hirschsprung's disease is rare and is excluded by a history of preceding normal bowel habit.
- Painful anal conditions often cause constipation.
- Where constipation is chronic, there will be acquired megacolon, and a need for prolonged treatment.
- Constipation with soiling is usually chronic, and treatment is not easy.
- Stool softeners (e.g. lactulose) regulate consistency; stimulants (e.g. senna) control frequency.

Useful literature

- The bowel habit of young children, L. Weaver and H. Steiner (*Archives of diseases in childhood*, vol. 59, pp. 649–52, 1984)
- Constipation, G. Clayden. In: *Recent advances in paediatrics* 9, T. David (ed.) (Churchill Livingstone, 1991)
- Preliminary report: the antegrade continence enema, P. Malone, P. Ransley and E. Kiely (*Lancet*, vol. 336, pp. 1217–18, 1990)
- *Constipation in childhood*, G. Clayden and S. Agnarsson (Oxford University Press, 1991)

24 Cystic fibrosis outpatient management

Cystic fibrosis affects approximately 1 in 2000 white children. Initially the domain of the general paediatrician, the care of children with cystic fibrosis has more recently been centred in regional clinics specifically for children with cystic fibrosis. It seems likely that specialised clinics improve the quality of care, as they allow a multidisciplinary evaluation and the development of expertise by doctors with a special interest in the condition. Specialist centres have the disadvantage of requiring patients to travel longer distances for both inpatient and outpatient care and more recently concern has been voiced regarding the problem of cross infection with both *Pseudomonas aeruginosa* and *Pseudomonas cepacia*. It seems likely, therefore, that local paediatric services will have some role in the ongoing care of children with cystic fibrosis, preferably sharing care with one of the larger centres. The aim of outpatient review is to monitor the child's condition, compliance with treatment and the need for change in treatment. The visit to the clinic will, moreover, offer moral support.

History

This is best taken by system.

Respiratory

Enquire as to the presence, frequency and nature of cough. If there is sputum, enquire as to the volume, colour and consistency. Is there dyspnoea on effort or exercise-induced wheeze or cough? Nasal obstruction may indicate either rhinitis or polyps.

Digestive

Enquire as to the appetite, stool frequency and colour. In infants there may also be a rectal prolapse and in adolescence symptoms of meconium ileus equivalent, such as colicky abdominal pain.

Miscellaneous

Joint problems or symptoms related to excess salt loss in sweat (particularly in warm climates) and symptoms related to liver decompensation.

Treatment

Enquire as to the use of pancreatic extract, the frequency and timing of dosage. Ask the patient to describe the daily routine of physiotherapy, nebulised bronchodilators or antibiotics and to demonstrate the inhaler technique where a device is being used. Ensure appropriate immunisation has been given (e.g. influenza vaccine).

Examination

Assessment of growth is perhaps the single most useful part of the clinical examination. Measure the height, weight and head circumference. Nutrition can be further assessed by measuring skinfold thickness over the triceps and subscapular areas. The mid arm circumference will give valuable information as to muscle bulk. Skinfold thickness measurement by callipers are subject to large interobserver variation and the measurements are best done by the same person at each clinic. Failure to sustain normal growth or a fall off in nutritional indices would imply a serious problem with either caloric intake, absorption or chest infection.

Look for clubbing and document severity. Is there any chest

deformity or accessory muscle usage? Objectively document hyperinflation by measuring chest circumference and the level of liver dullness. Auscultation is part of the clinical routine but is a rather blunt instrument in assessing children with cystic fibrosis. The chest may sound very clear in the presence of considerable airways disease and this is probably due to a widespread airway plugging which prevents sounds being conducted to the chest wall. On abdominal examination, look specifically for evidence of liver enlargement or hardness and splenic enlargement. Children with meconium ileus equivalent may have a mass palpable in the right iliac fossa. Infants with poorly controlled malabsorption may have perianal excoriation due to sugar in the stools and also rectal prolapse where nutrition is poor. Examination of the ears and nose is important to seek evidence of glue ear and nasal polyps.

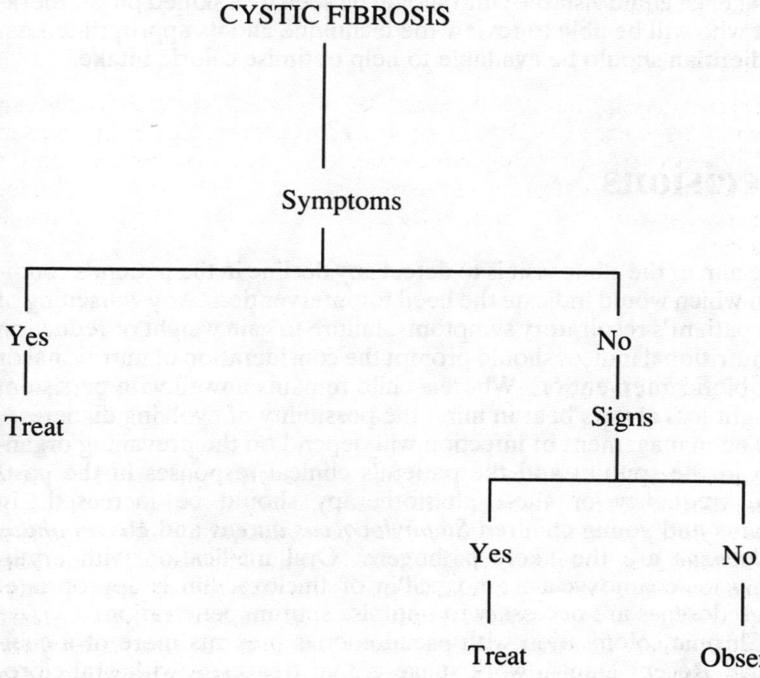

Fig. 24.1 Pathway for outpatient surveillance of cystic fibrosis

Laboratory data

Regular measurement of lung function is mandatory. Simple measurement of forced expiratory volume in one second and oxygen saturation should be possible at most outpatient visits with periodic full evaluations of flow volume loop. Chest X-rays should be performed at least annually and as otherwise indicated by the clinical condition. Regular monitoring of sputum culture is perhaps the single most useful test. Infants and young children will rarely provide sputum and in these circumstances a cough swab may be useful. In older children, colonised with pseudomonas, there may be poor agreement between laboratory culture and sensitivity reports and the clinical response to antibiotics. On an annual basis it is reasonable to check levels of the fat soluble vitamins, liver function tests and to look for evidence of occult diabetes mellitus, particularly in older children.

At each clinic visit the child should be seen by a skilled physiotherapist who will be able to review the technique and its appropriateness. A dietitian should be available to help optimise calorie intake.

Decisions

The aim of the clinic visit is to detect any decline in the patient's condition which would indicate the need for intervention. Any worsening of the patient's respiratory symptoms, failure to gain weight or reduction in nutritional indices should prompt the consideration of nutritional or antibiotic intervention. Where a child remains unwell with persistent weight loss always bear in mind the possibility of evolving diabetes.

The management of infection will depend on the prevailing organism in the sputum and the patient's clinical responses in the past. The frequency of chest physiotherapy should be increased. In infants and young children *Staphylococcus aureus* and *Haemophilus influenzae* are the likely pathogens. Oral medication with erythromycin, coamoxyclav, amoxycillin or flucloxacillin is appropriate. High dosages are necessary to optimise sputum penetration.

Chronic colonisation with pseudomonas presents more of a challenge. Recent Danish work suggests that treatment with oral ciprofloxacin and nebulised colomicin, given when pseudomonas is first cultured in sputum, may prevent or delay chronic colonisation. Ciprofloxacin is an orally administered antipseudomonal agent, but the organisms frequently develop resistance. Nebulised antibiotics are an option and where these are used, attention to detail is important with nebuliser usage and servicing. Gentamicin and colomicin are the most commonly used antibiotics and more recently, tobramycin in high dosage has been found to be useful. Where symptoms progress despite oral and nebulised treatment, a course of intravenous treatment is necessary. Comparative clinical trials are distinctly scarce and practice is usually informed by experience and personal bias. It is generally agreed that at least two weeks of antibiotic treatment should be given and most clinicians prefer a combination of a cephalosporin or semisynthetic penicillin with aminoglycide; combinations such as ceftazidime and gentamicin, piperacillin and gentamicin, azlocillin and tobramycin all have their advocates.

Nutrition intervention is indicated where there is clear evidence of malabsorption. This may declare itself clinically with obvious steatorrhoea or on a more sophisticated assessment such as measurement of fecal fat output. In general, it is best for children to have a normal diet, with supplements added, rather than taking a large part of their calories as high density carbohydrates. Pancreatic enzymes should be given in an enteric coating, in doses adequate to prevent diarrhoea and optimise weight gain. High dose preparations may cause colonic strictures. More invasive nutritional support such as nocturnal nasogastric feeds or (percutaneous endoscopic) gastrostomy feeds are best left to the specialist centres.

Children with cystic fibrosis have asthma at least as frequently as the rest of the population and it is important that this is considered and adequately treated.

Much of the lung damage in CF is mediated by the host's own neutrophil elastase. The role of oral steroids in management remains controversial. The initial suggestion that administration of prednisolone 2 mg/kg on alternative days improved outcome has been offset by an unacceptably high rate of side effects. The value of lower doses of oral or high dose inhaled steroids is being evaluated. Specific anti elastase agents are not yet available.

The median survival for children with cystic fibrosis has increased steadily over the past two decades. This has been achieved largely through meticulous attention to the minor details of treatment. There is realistic hope that more specific treatment will be available in the near future. The role of newer agents such as amiloride, DNase and ursodeoxycholic acid (for hepatic problems) remains to be established.

Key points

- Most children with CF have near normal lifestyle.
- Compliance with regular chest physiotherapy is essential.
- The improved outlook for CF is due to meticulous application of simple principles.
- Pseudomonas colonisation may be eradicated if treated early.
- New treatments hold the promise of further improvements in prognosis.

Useful literature

- *The diagnosis and management of paediatric respiratory disease,* R. Dinwiddie (Churchill Livingstone, 1990)

25 Developmental delay

A large number of children are referred to paediatric clinics for an opinion as to whether their development is normal or not. Another significant number of children are being followed up because of possible concerns about their future development, for example survivors of neonatal care. This chapter is written to help in deciding which children have significant delay, of what type and what investigations should be performed. The management of these children will depend

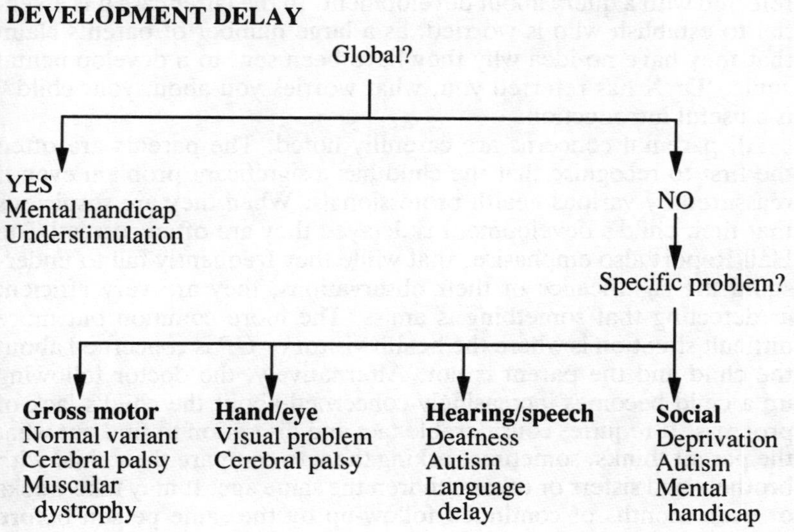

Fig. 25.1 Diagnostic pathway for developmental delay

on local provisions and further guidance should be sought from a senior colleague.

Developmental examination tends to be poorly performed in DCH and membership examination, possibly reflecting on the SHOs' teaching, but with a greater involvement of GPs in developmental surveillance and increased access to developmental courses, the situation is rightfully changing. It is essential to know the normal and there is a lot to learn by testing the development of children that are admitted for elective procedures.

There are a number of books which are essential reading. The Hall Report questions the whole value of developmental surveillance but emphasises the importance of listening to parents. Normal development is well covered by Illingworth, Sheridan and Bax. Whilst the important investigations are discussed, the reader is referred to Stevenson and King for a complete summary (see Useful literature).

History

The child will either be attending follow-up clinic or will have been referred with a query about development. In the latter case it is essential to establish who is worried, as a large number of parents claim that they have no idea why they have been sent to a developmental clinic. 'Dr X has referred you, what worries you about your child?' is a useful introduction.

All parental concerns are carefully noted. The parents are often the first to recognise that the child has a significant problem even if reassured by various health professionals. When they are suspicious that their child's development is delayed they are often correct! The Hall Report also emphasises that while they frequently fail to understand the significance of their observations, they are very efficient at detecting that something is amiss. The more common but more difficult situation is where the health visitor or GP is concerned about the child and the parent is not. Alternatively, the doctor following up a child becomes increasingly concerned about the child's lack of progress. It requires considerable tact and discretion to find out what the parent thinks, sometimes asking them to compare their child with brothers and sisters or other children the same age. It may take weeks or even months of continued follow-up by the same person before the parents agree that there is a problem. After a full description of the concern it is sensible to take a full developmental history. The majority of children referred will be in the preschool age group.

Development can be divided into four main areas:

1. posture and gross motor
2. vision and fine motor
3. hearing and speech
4. social behaviour and play.

It is often useful to establish the developmental sequence in each of these areas, perhaps beginning with the area that the parent is most concerned about. With a younger child questions can be asked about development with time. It is vitally important that both doctor and parent understand each other. 'When did he smile?' means 'when did he smile in response to a face' not 'when did he smile with wind'. It is important to note that the child is continuing to make developmental progress, albeit slowly, to exclude the rare but genetically important regressive conditions. Note any parental concerns regarding hearing or vision.

It is essential to document the child's early feeding, time of first smile, ability to chew solids and when the child stopped deliberately throwing objects to the floor. There are surprising similarities in the histories of children who have significant developmental delay. They may have been difficult feeders or alternatively are described as 'perfect' babies – 'you never knew they were there'. There is often a history that they slept for long periods as babies and infants. In significant global delay, all milestones are delayed. Many milestones have large normal variations, but smiling is relatively fixed at 4–6 weeks of age and delayed smiling at 3 or 4 months may be the first sign of a problem delay. Chewing usually begins at 6–8 months and delay may cause vomiting and feeding difficulties. Taking everything to the mouth is normal at 6–12 months, but may be prolonged for two or three years in children with severe learning difficulties. Deliberate throwing of objects on the floor usually stops by 15 or 16 months but also persists in children with significant problems.

In a full history it is essential to note the details of pregnancy including any admissions, bleeding, drugs or X-rays. The maternal age at delivery and past obstetric history including miscarriages must be noted. A family history of similar problems or consanguinity must be sought.

Examination

This will begin by watching the child coming into the clinic room. As the initial history is being taken the child should be observed playing with a small number of toys that are there to 'warm the child up' prior to a developmental examination. It is vitally important to observe the child's interest in surroundings and concentration on tasks. When the initial history is taken and before the child gets bored developmental examinations should begin. For toddlers, it is better to have the child seated at a small table close to the mother. A number of techniques can be used. For the novice the repeated use of developmental tests such as the Denver will teach confidence. Alternatively, the methods of Illingworth or Sheridan can be followed. There is a lot of common ground between these and all rely on simple apparatus such as cubes, pencil, form boards, etc. It is essential to engage the child's interest and the cubes are often useful as a starter for this. Once interest is lost the item is withdrawn and a new one quickly substituted. The advantage of the Denver screen is that the tests to be done are described with their normal variations and they can quickly be recorded as pass, fail or reported by parent. Again it is crucial to emphasise that it is not simply what the child achieves, but his interest and his way of achieving it that is important.

Physical examination

The height, weight and head circumference must be recorded and plotted. A small head (microcephaly) is a significant indicator of a small brain. A careful search must be made for dysmorphic features, noting if these are also present in the parents. A full neurological examination must be performed. Vision must be tested before hearing. If there is any parental concern about hearing or language, the hearing must be checked if the doctor is adequately trained in audiological techniques. If not, they should be referred to the local audiological service or community clinic.

Management

The initial decision must be whether the child is within the normal range or whether the child's development is suspect. It cannot be overemphasised that even the most experienced observer may be unable to establish for certain whether a child will have significant problems in the future. Illingworth has given many examples of mistakes that even he has made. The most important investigation is repeated assessment of the child's development over time. The areas of development that cause concern to parents and doctors can be discussed, but a diagnosis of developmental delay or a specific problem such as cerebral palsy should only be made when an experienced doctor is as certain as he can be that his diagnosis is true.

Investigation and management of significant developmental delay must deal with the parents' four questions:

- What is wrong?
- Why did it happen?
- Can it happen again? (in a subsequent pregnancy)
- What is the plan?

If the child's development is suspect the next decision is to see if the child is globally delayed or if the child has a significant problem in one area of development (Fig. 25.1). The term mental retardation (IQ less than 70) is gradually being replaced by the term learning difficulties. To make such a diagnosis, the child's development must be significantly behind in all areas of development. The younger these children present, the more likely they are to have serious delay. Suspecting a problem and investigating it is just one part of the prolonged multidisciplinary involvement that these children need. In all global delay it is essential to establish whether there might be any degree of social understimulation.

Investigations depend on the whole clinical picture but will include karyotype (fragile X analysis must be specifically requested if suspected), creatinine kinase and an amino acid profile. An EEG may sometimes show undetected seizures. For a full discussion see Stevenson and King.

The developmental profile may show a marked delay in one area of development or alternatively the child is globally delayed but more severely in some areas. A common cause for concern by doctor and parent is delay in motor development. The concern is usually that the child is not sitting or not walking. Failure to sit or bear weight at six months is common, but sitting balance is usually achieved by nine months. In the case of perceived motor delay additional questions should be asked about the motor development of siblings and importantly of the parents themselves. An important familial variant of normal is bottom shuffling. This often causes delay in walking to 18 months. It is important to consider cerebral palsy and muscular dystrophy.

The diagnosis of cerebral palsy is difficult, particularly in the first year of life. It should not be based on the presence of brisk reflexes, but on the observation of an abnormal and delayed pattern of movement. As with global delay, repeated observation is usually necessary before a definitive diagnosis can be given to the parents. Warning signs for hemiplegia include obvious hand preference in the first year of life, the gross motor abilities may be normal or mildly delayed but the crawl will be asymmetrical. The lateral and forward parachutes will be absent on the affected side. With spastic diplegia, the legs will be stiff and it may be noted that it is difficult to change the nappy and that the baby kicks both legs together – reciprocal kicking. It is important to check the tone at the ankles and hips and to look for a 'catch' when the hips are quickly abducted. In quadriplegia there is often associated global delay with or without convulsions. Duchenne muscular dystrophy, although rare, is important to diagnose so that parents can be advised about the risk to any future children.

Delays in fine motor ability in younger children are uncommon and may be the first signs of hemiplegia. With severe visual problems there is often a delay in gross motor ability as well as fine motor function. Specific problems in speech and language are common, particularly in boys aged 3–4 years. Any child with a language problem must have their hearing checked. A clinical decision must be made as to whether this is a delay in comprehension, expression or both. Referral to a speech therapist is often indicated. An important point about investigation is that children with significant language delay should be tested to exclude fragile X and muscular dystrophy, since these may present with the language problem before the motor disability is recognised.

Language problems may co-exist with delays in social abilities in the case of autism. These children may have good non-verbal abilities with items such as puzzles, but show absolutely no interest in anyone in the room. It can often be extremely difficult to differentiate this condition from specific language problems and an extended period of multidisciplinary assessments is often required.

Summary

It is essential to know the normal child development and its variants. Children with suspected developmental delay must be followed up and the most important investigation is their progress over time. If a child's development is suspect guidance from a senior colleague is essential. Further management of significantly delayed children is usually supervised by a multidisciplinary team working in a child development centre.

Key points

- The range of normal developmental (especially motor) progression is wide.
- The damage of inappropriate diagnosis may outweigh the advantages of any intervention.
- Where delay is global – simple mental handicap or neglect is likely.
- Where delay is in a single area of development – a specific cause is likely.
- It is difficult (and may be inadvisable) to diagnose cerebral palsy in the first year.
- Deafness is the most important cause of speech delay.
- Repeated assessment after an interval is the most valuable investigation.

Useful literature

- *Health for all children. A programme for child health surveillance*, 2nd edition, D. Hall (Oxford University Press, 1991)
- *The development of the infant and young child; normal and abnormal*, R. Illingworth (Churchill Livingstone, 1987)
- *Basic developmental screening 0–4 years*, R. Illingworth (Blackwell, 1988)
- *Child development and child health*, M. Bax, H. Hart and S. Jenkins (Blackwell, 1990)
- *Handbook of neurological investigations in children*, J. Stevenson and M. King (Wright, 1989)
- The Denver II: A major revision and restandardisation of the Denver Developmental Screening Test, W. Frankenburg, J. Dodds, P. Archer *et al.* (*Pediatrics*, vol. 89, pp. 91–7, 1992)

26 Diabetes mellitus outpatient management

Introduction

With a prevalence of between 1 and 2 per 1000 children, diabetes mellitus is one of the commoner chronic illnesses of childhood. It is unlikely that any individual general practitioner would have sufficient caseload to generate the necessary expertise, so that childhood diabetes is best supervised in the hospital outpatient setting. The aims of outpatient care of diabetes are to allow the patient to have a normal childhood whilst avoiding the immediate and long-term complications of diabetes. Complications would include short-term hypoglycaemia and ketoacidosis. Retinopathy, nephropathy, neuropathy and vascular disease are the major long-term complications and are delayed or prevented by the maintenance of normoglycaemia in adults. Glycaemic control in the prepubertal period seems to have only a minor influence on the development of long-term complications. Therefore intensive insulin regimes, with their attendant risk of hypoglycaemia which may be fatal or impair brain development, are inappropriate in young children. During and after puberty, diabetes care should strive for near normoglycaemia. It is best to talk of 'children with diabetes' rather than 'diabetics'.

History

Enquiry as to general well-being and any recent health problems is a useful introduction. Enquire specifically as to whether there has been any significant hypoglycaemia or difficulties with metabolic control. Compliance with diet is often a problem but this is lessened when the whole family adopt the same diet. The 'diary card' often forms a central part of the consultation. If the clinician is not sensitive to the patient's needs, the diary can become part of an elaborate game. Children rarely measure their blood sugar as frequently as doctors think and trying to trap them will give the wrong message. It is best to regard the diary card as the patient's record which will assist him and his parents in making any necessary adjustments. Do not look at the diary card as a routine, only when invited to by the parents and the child or if there is a specific problem.

Ask the child how much insulin he is taking. As a rough guide, in the first year after diagnosis the average dose of insulin should be approximately 0.5 units per kg per day, increasing to 1 unit per kg per day after a year and peaking at approximately 1.5 units per kg per day at times of rapid growth, e.g. early infancy or puberty. An insulin dose that has not varied for several months or is very different from the anticipated levels above should be a cause for concern. The doctor needs to know the preparations and delivery systems for insulin. Pre-mixed combinations given with a "pen" are the most popular.

Clinical examination

Measurement of height and weight is essential. Failure to achieve normal linear growth and weight gain implies poor metabolic control. Excessive weight gain indicates that both calorie intake and insulin dosage are too high.

Measure the blood pressure. Inspect the injection sites and palpate the areas generally to see if there is any lipohypertrophy. A cursory glance at the fingertips will help give the clinician an idea as to the frequency of blood sugar monitoring. Examination of the fundi should be routine in children over the age of 12 years. (Retinopathy does not occur before puberty.)

Laboratory data

Measurements of glycosylated haemoglobin correlates crudely with the maintenance of normoglycaemia. The aim is to achieve levels of less than one and a half times the mean for the non-diabetic population. Annual measurement of serum lipids is worthwhile. The measurement of urinary microalbuminuria in childhood is controversial, but in adulthood would seem to be cost effective. Treatment with captopril seems to slow progression of nephropathy.

Decisions

The aim of the consultation is to decide whether there should be an alteration in the monitoring, the dosage and timing of insulin or the dietary prescription. Decisions are best taken jointly with the patient and the parents and will need to be accompanied by further education. Patient education in diabetes is a continuous process and carries on for many years after diagnosis. Emotional and behavioural problems are common, particularly in the wake of diagnosis and during adolescence. Patience and empathy are prerequisites for successful management and even with these, there will be periods where patient behaviour defies rational explanation!

Families should have access to a social worker, and dietician. The nurse specialist in diabetes has been a welcome addition to diabetes care. Parents and children may find the nurse less intimidating, more accessible and approachable than their doctor.

Our primary aim in management of diabetes in children is to enable them to enjoy a normal childhood whilst developing good habits and attitudes that will enable them to successfully manage their diabetes and lessen the risk of the more severe long-term complications.

Key points

- Tight glycaemic control before puberty is difficult, may be dangerous, and does not reduce the risks of complications.
- Insulin requirements are usually 0.5 unit/kg/day for the year after diagnosis, then 1.0 unit/kg/day increasing to 1.5 unit/kg/day at times of rapid growth during puberty.
- Transfer management to the child before puberty.
- Maintenance of near normoglycaemia from puberty onward reduces the risk of long-term complications.

Useful literature

- *Care of the child with diabetes*, J. Baum and A Kinmonth (Churchill Livingstone, 1985).

27 Nocturnal enuresis

Introduction

Enuresis is a symptom, not a disorder or a condition. It causes considerable discomfort, some disability and a lot of dissatisfaction for parents and children. Enuresis is involuntary micturition in bed at night beyond an age when it ceases to be acceptable behaviour. This is usually taken to be five years. About 90 per cent of children achieve dryness at 5 years. The recognition and definition of nocturnal enuresis as a problem will vary amongst practitioners. It is reasonable to define it as a problem when it occurs sufficiently frequently to upset the child and concern the mother. Bedwetting is commoner in boys, in the less well off and in urban children. The prevalence of enuresis is approximately 10 per cent amongst 5-year-olds, 5 per cent amongst 10-year-olds and 1 per cent amongst 15-year-olds (Fig. 27.1). There is a spontaneous resolution rate of 15 per cent per annum independent of any treatment effect. There are few good data pertaining to adults, but anecdotal reports suggest that enuresis can persist in adulthood, sometimes intermittent (with alcohol ingestion) and occasionally continuous.

Enuresis is best divided into primary (where a child has never achieved consistent dryness) and secondary (where a child has been reliably dry and relapses). Primary enuresis accounts for approximately 75 per cent of presentations.

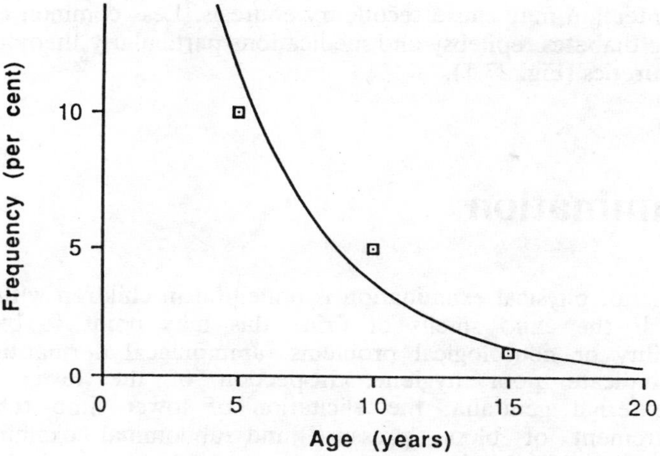

Fig. 27.1 Spontaneous resolution of bed-wetting

History

The history will attempt to define whether the enuresis is primary or secondary, to exclude 'organic' causes and uncover aggravating factors. Age, sex and rank in family are relevant. Where enuresis is primary the absence of daytime symptoms and the achievement of at least some dry nights provides strong assurance as to the absence of organic disease. Conversely, continuous wetting and daytime problems may indicate neurological or urological problems. Domestic sleeping arrangements, toilet facilities and home stability are all important. There is often a strong family history amongst children with primary enuresis. It is important to ascertain the parents' reaction to the enuresis, whether this is punitive or whether they have resorted to putting the child in nappies again. The child's behaviour whilst away from home may provide valuable clues. Try to ascertain which measures and treatments have been previously tried and assess compliance with these.

Where enuresis is secondary try to define whether there was an associated precipitating event, such as commencement of school, birth of a new sibling, moving home, parental absence, illness, disharmony or financial problems. The age at which dryness was achieved and the ease with which this was attained are also relevant. Urinary tract infection may cause secondary enuresis. Less common causes include diabetes, epilepsy and medications particularly theophylline and diuretics (Fig. 27.1).

Examination

In general, physical examination is unhelpful in children with enuresis. If the child smells of urine this may point to bladder instability or neurological problems; ammoniacal dermatitis will also indicate poor hygiene. Inspection of the lower spine and external genitalia, the elicitation of lower limb reflexes, measurement of blood pressure and abdominal examination looking specifically for the presence of bladder dullness are all mandatory. If there is any suspicion of child sexual abuse a careful 'forensic' examination is important. Constipation may predispose to urinary infection and indirectly be responsible for nocturnal enuresis.

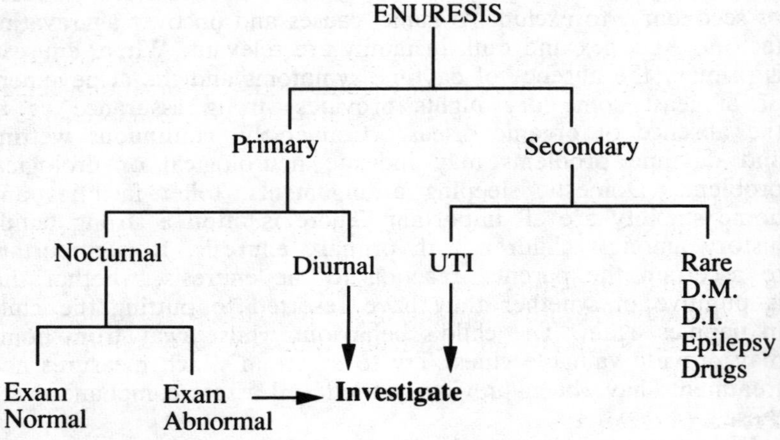

Fig. 27.2 Assessment pathway for enuresis

Evaluation

Based on the history and examination it should be possible to categorise enuresis as:

Primary: Benign
Organic

Secondary: Stress related
Organic

Organic associations with enuresis are uncommon. Testing the urine for the presence of sugar or infection is reasonable in secondary enuresis. Detailed neurological or urodynamic evaluation is indicated where clues in the history or the examination would point towards the possibility of spinal cord disease or bladder muscle inco-ordination.

Management

Most children who wet their beds can be managed by their primary physician. The most important aspects of management at all ages include:

- Good doctoring (demonstrating an interest, being enthusiastic).
- Sympathetic interview of parent and child. It is sometimes helpful to interview together and then separately. Older children must be allowed to give their version of the problem.
- Reassurance of normality.
- Setting reasonable targets.
- Being positive – record only dry nights and give rewards for success.
- Regular follow-up every 4–8 weeks.
- Avoiding negative approaches. If enuresis is soluble with praise, it surely and certainly worsens with criticism and shame.

Preschool children

Usually little intervention is necessary. If previously dry try re-education with positive reinforcement. Avoid the use of nappies if the child objects to them. If there are also daytime symptoms, concentrate on these initially.

Aged 5–7 years

Follow the simple guidelines above – praise, positive attitude, patience, perseverance and a few pennies! Set simple dryness goals and foster a positive attitude by stressing the dry nights. Children of this age revel in praise. Star charts are simple and supportive, but can sometimes be distressing if they merely reinforce the child's lack of progress; timing is important! Fluid restriction is more harmful than helpful, since denial of drinks creates conflicts which we are trying to avoid. Lifting the child, as the parents retire, may help. Obvious psychosocial problems need to be addressed. In the older child if simple measures fail, and the child is motivated, a buzzer alarm can be tried.

Aged 8–10 years

It is reasonable to try an enuretic alarm in the first instance. There are several types and time must be taken explaining the operation, care and possible problems of these devices. They are relatively expensive but effective and are perhaps not as widely used as they ought to be. Unfortunately some children, who appear to sleep deeply, do not awake through the alarm noise and may need a parent near by to stir them from their slumbers.

Aged 11–15 years

At this stage many manoeuvres will have been tried and failed. A thorough reappraisal of the problem and perhaps a second opinion is advisable. Buzzer alarms can be very effective in this age group if compliance is good. Exploration of family dynamics and perhaps psychological or child psychiatry assessment may be indicated.

Drug treatments

The road to nocturnal dryness is littered with discarded drugs. They can occasionally be employed as a 'crutch' to achieve short-term dryness, but are not effective as a 'cure'. With all drugs there is a relatively high relapse rate on withdrawal. The major medications used are the tricyclic antidepressants and synthetic antidiuretic hormone. Imipramine is said to work on the basis of its anticholinergic activity and perhaps some modification of sleep pattern. It must not be forgotten that tricyclic antidepressants are very dangerous if taken in excessive dosage. Desmopressin works by reducing nocturnal urine production, but does not address the problem of why these children do not wake up when their bladder is full! Whilst desmopressin is perhaps more physiological, it is much more expensive than imipramine. Desmopressin is useful for achieving short-term dryness and in primary nocturnal enuresis resistant to alarms and other manoeuvres.

Key points

- Above all, be enthusiastic and empathic.
- If you or a parent or a colleague wet when younger share this secret with the enuretic child. James Joyce, John Osborne and Barbra Streisand are amongst some of the notable sufferers!
- Evaluate the frequency of enuresis for 4–6 weeks before initiating any action. Merely showing an interest is often therapeutic.
- Don't be deterred by mother saying 'we tried that before'. A third party might succeed where parents have failed.
- It is possible to resolve the symptom of enuresis without alleviating the apparent cause.
- Remember that children are a very good barometer of the familial emotional climate. Enuresis which fails to resolve merits deeper exploration of the family interaction.

Useful literature

- Establishment of working definitions in nocturnal enuresis, R. Butler (*Archives of diseases in childhood*, vol. 66, pp. 267–71, 1991)
- Nocturnal enuresis: epidemiology, evaluation, and currently available treatment options, H. Rushton (*Journal of paediatrics*, vol. 114, p. 691–6, 1989)
- 50 years of enuretic alarms, W. Forsythe and R. Butler (*Archives of diseases in childhood*, vol. 64, pp. 879–85, 1989)

28 Failure to thrive

Introduction

Failure to thrive describes failure to gain weight normally. This clinical problem is most common in the first two years of life when the rate of weight gain is maximal and linear growth is largely determined by nutrition rather than hormonal influences. In later childhood, linear growth is determined by growth hormone, thyroxine and the sex hormones, the presentation of failure to thrive is less common and the causes are dominantly nutritional, e.g. anorexia nervosa, Crohn's disease, malabsorption. Implicit in the clinical presentation is the documentation of failure to gain weight. This implies serial measures which have indicated poor growth, rather than a single measure which will merely indicate 'size'.

Normal growth requires stable external and internal (bodily) environments, normal nutritional intake, digestion, absorption and utilisation. Disturbance of any of these processes may result in failure to thrive. Accordingly the causes of failure to thrive can be broadly categorised into:

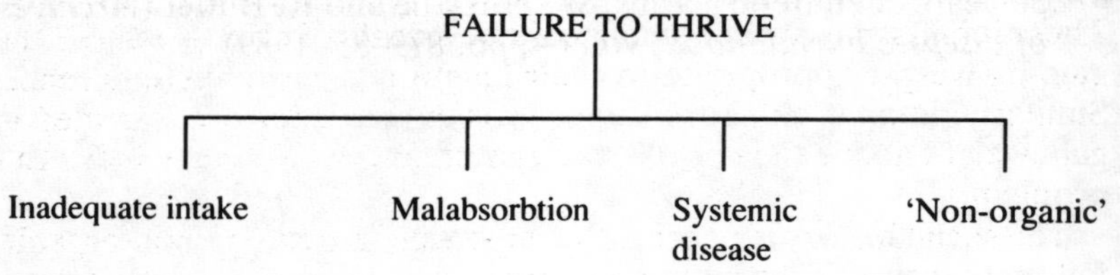

Fig. 28.1 Diagnostic possibilities in failure to thrive

1. inadequate intake,
2. inadequate absorption,
3. systemic illness, and
4. social or non-organic causes.

History

A clear documentation of the age of onset of the problem and events surrounding onset is necessary. What symptoms encouraged the parents to attend their doctor? Failure to gain weight may be part of a constellation of symptoms which will point to an obvious cause. Where symptoms are not specifically volunteered key items to be elicited concern the child's appetite, any vomiting, the bowel habit and the child's level of activity. Obtain an accurate history of the feeding pattern. 'Unsuccessful' breastfeeding is a common cause of failure to thrive and often occurs where the mother is malnourished, unsupported or inexperienced. Where artificial feeds are used, clearly document the method of reconstitution, the volume and frequency of feeds. The time at which solid feeds are introduced and particularly the timing of the introduction of wheat or gluten containing feeds are important.

In the past history previous intestinal surgery would clearly be important. Major gut resection, particularly where the ileocaecal valve has been removed, may well result in 'short-gut' syndrome. Recurrent illnesses, such as respiratory tract infection, may in themselves cause failure to thrive or may point towards an underlying condition such as cystic fibrosis. Similarly, urinary infection may be clinically silent but can give rise to failure to thrive, particularly if there is coexistent renal insufficiency.

The effects of pregnancy are also important, since this may colour the clinical evaluation. For instance, the infant of a diabetic mother may be macrosomic and fail to gain weight relative to the birthweight. These infants may appear to fail to thrive transiently but usually settle, gaining weight appropriate to their length and head circumference. Similarly, infants with intrauterine growth restriction are expected to gain weight above the normal rate and failure to do so may indicate a problem.

The social history is particularly important in cases of 'non-organic' failure to thrive. If the mother is young, socially isolated or depressed, the child may lack the necessary security and affection to thrive normally. Equally, an unstable, violent and chaotic home background can have a similar effect. Non-organic failure to thrive is commoner in the firstborn children and also if there has been a long gap between children – the 'afterthought'. Worldwide, simple poverty is commonest cause of the failure to thrive.

In the family history, try to document parental size as this may indicate a constitutionally small background, but would not explain a failure to gain weight at the normal rate. The presence of familial illnesses such as coeliac disease and cystic fibrosis should be sought.

Examination

The most important part of examination is simple measurement. Accurately measure the child's height, weight and head circumference and plot these on percentile charts that are appropriate for the child's race, country of origin and, where relevant, specific syndrome, e.g. Down's syndrome or Turner syndrome. Always allow for the effect of extreme prematurity, certainly until the child is over two years of age. Measurements at a single time point will indicate whether the child is symmetrically small or has asymmetric growth, i.e. the weight is disparately low for the height and head circumference percentiles.

A 'symmetrically' small child will have height, weight and head circumference of similarly low percentile values and this would tend to indicate either a constitutional problem or else severe, perhaps prenatal, nutritional problems. 'Asymmetric' failure to gain weight usually implies a nutritional aetiology. Accuracy of measurements is absolutely vital, particularly where serial measurements are being used to assess growth velocity. Attention to simple details is important, but all too often forgotten. Serial measurements,with plotting on appropriate centile charts, will allow a clear documentation of either appropriate weight gain or failure to thrive.

Clinical examination should always include measurement of the blood pressure (children with chronic renal failure may otherwise appear completely normal). A clinical assessment of nutrition is always important. The axilla and the groin area should usually have ample subcutaneous fat; if there appears to be redundant skin then the child is undernourished. If your clinical assessment of nutrition disagrees with the measurements; your eyes are usually correct.

Carefully assess the child for any dysmorphic features which may suggest syndromic growth restriction. A general examination should exclude systemic causes of failure to thrive. Where heart failure is causing the problem there should be evidence of tachypnoea, tachycardia, hepatomegaly with or without a murmur. A chronic respiratory problem may be evidenced by the presence of clubbing, tachypnoea, recession or signs on auscultation. Abdominal examination should seek evidence of hepatomegaly, splenomegaly, renal masses or a mass in the right iliac fossa which might indicate Crohn's disease. Neurological causes of failure to thrive will usually be clinically obvious but occasionally the 'diencephalic' syndrome may cause confusion with a relative absence of clinical signs in the presence of a cerebral tumour.

Assessment

On the basis of the history and examination it should be possible to categorise the child's problem and then to tailor investigation depending on the mechanism underlying growth failure (Fig. 28.1). In all cases where there is significant weight deficit it is prudent to check urine to exclude infection as this may be a clinically inapparent cause of growth failure.

Inadequate intake

Where the feeding history has documented a clearly inadequate intake or where the child is vomiting large quantities of the feed, simple attention to detail may sort out the problem. In the breastfeeding mother simple advice and support may ensure successful lactation but where the child's weight deficit is significant, complementary formula feeds should be offered after breastfeeds and the child observed closely to ensure adequate catch-up growth.

Malabsorption

This cause is suggested by a history of abnormal stool with diarrhoea or frank steatorrhoea . A simple stool test for sugar will indicate carbohydrate malabsorption; the presence of neutral fat in the stool suggests inadequate pancreatic function. In the smaller infant measurement of immunoreactive trypsin is a very useful screening test for cystic fibrosis. The sweat test provides a definitive diagnosis. Jejunal biopsy is indicated where there is a suspicion of coeliac disease. This can only be diagnosed after gluten has been introduced to the diet. More recently the finding of elevated IgA antigliaden antibodies in combination with particular HLA subtypes provides strong suggestive evidence for the diagnosis. A gluten free diet is curative but is necessary for life. Children with clinical coeliac disease are invariably miserable – 'the smiling, active child does not have coeliac disease'.

Systemic illness

Systemic illness as a cause of failure to thrive will usually be detected on clinical evaluation. Congenital heart disease causing failure to thrive usually does so via reduced intake of feed caused by breathlessness secondary to heart failure. Failure to thrive should not be ascribed to congenital heart disease which does not cause heart failure or cyanosis (such as a small ventricular septal defect). Chronic respiratory distress due to bronchopulmonary dysplasia, cystic fibrosis or other rare lung conditions may cause failure to thrive by increasing the work of breathing and causing chronic hypoxia. Liver failure may cause poor weight gain because of maldigestion of fats or through a non-specific effect on metabolism. Chronic renal insufficiency will cause restriction of linear growth as well as weight gain and may be a particularly difficult clinical problem in the absence of definitive treatment of the renal disorder. Children with severe mental and/or physical handicap often fail to thrive. This is due to a series of problems, commonly poor appetite, difficulty with chewing and swallowing, recurrent illness associated with immobility and complicating pulmonary and renal infections.

Non-organic or social causes

Non-organic or social causes of failure to thrive is often a diagnosis of exclusion. The family background may be suggestive but it is very important to exclude 'organic' causes. This may be a particularly difficult diagnosis and is often based on the response of the child's weight to admission to hospital or to foster care. Collateral information from the community health service and the general practitioner usually proves very helpful in suggesting and making the diagnosis.

Investigation

Investigations clearly depend on the clinical suspicion. Urgent investigation is indicated in the child who is ill, has sustained recent acute weight loss or in whom the diagnosis is unclear. A useful screen would consist of a full blood count, full serum biochemical profile including a venous pH, a chest X-ray, a mid-stream specimen of urine, and stool examination for the presence of ova, parasites, fat and sugar. Management of the problem will be directed to the cause. In many cases no clear aetiology is identified and children appear to recover on follow-up. It is unfortunate that this group of children have clearly not read the paediatric texts but they do exist and one must accept that a diagnostic failure and a well child are not mutually exclusive.

Key points

- Serial measurement is necessary to define failure to thrive.
- Unsuccessful lactation is the most common cause in infancy.
- Malabsorption is usually evident from the history.
- Many cases defy categorisation and improve spontaneously.
- Most cases can be investigated and managed as outpatients.

Useful literature

- Failure to thrive, H. Marcovitch (*British medical journal*, 1994, 308, 35–3)

29 Fits and funny turns

Introduction

A fit (or convulsion or seizure) is an episode of abnormal involuntary motor activity primarily due to abnormal electrochemical activity in the brain. There is usually loss of consciousness. Seizures may occur with serious metabolic disturbance, systemic illness and particularly brain injury. In some children seizure occurs without obvious cause.

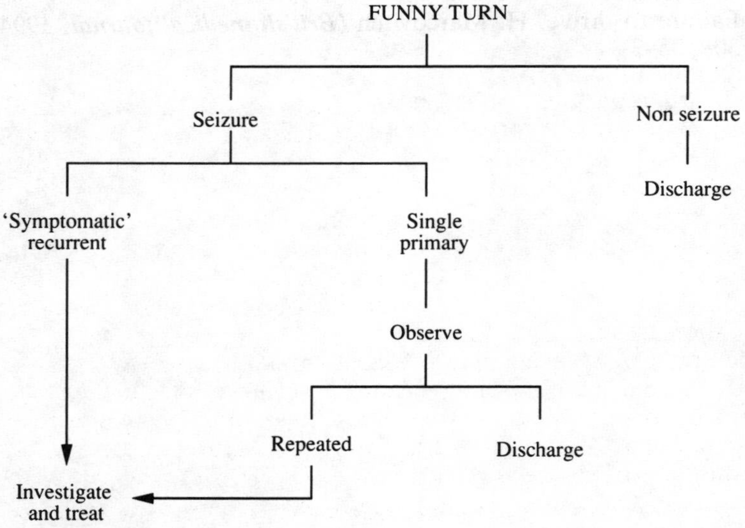

Fig. 29.1 Management pathway for 'funny turns'

A febrile convulsion is a fit, triggered by fever, in a child aged 6 months to 5 years. Some 3–5 per cent of children have febrile convulsions, and these recur in one third.

Epilepsy is a condition which is characterised by recurrent afebrile seizures. Less than 1 per cent of children are affected. Epilepsy is best considered as either symptomatic (a symptom of brain injury) or idiopathic (where brain structure and function are normal). The prognosis for the latter is good.

A 'funny turn' describes unusual episodic behaviour which may be confused with a seizure. Funny turns are far more common than seizures and give rise to much parental anxiety.

Careful history is the most valuable technique for differentiating fits and funny turns. Where epilepsy is excluded, much anxiety will be removed. If epilepsy is diagnosed a positive attitude is appropriate, since control with safe medication is usually possible and the prognosis for remission is good. The word 'epileptic' should never be used to describe people with epilepsy.

History

A clear history from a reliable witness provides the most useful diagnostic information. Carefully document preceding events, any prodrome and the sequential evolution of the episode. Pay particular attention to any suggestion of focal onset with secondary generalisation. In doubtful cases, the presence of incontinence or tongue/cheek injury may be a useful indicator of genuine seizure. The description of the seizure may be diagnostic. Awareness is usually clouded, but may be retained in a focal seizure. 'Absences' lasting for a few seconds with occasional automatisms are usually due to petit mal. Longer periods of absence may indicate temporal lobe epilepsy. Generalised 'grand mal' seizures have an initial tonic phase where there is generalised stiffening with tongue biting, incontinence and often a cry; the clonic phase then ensues.

The timing of the event may give clues – prolonged fast may suggest hypoglycaemia. Early morning seizures are also typical of benign focal epilepsy. Nocturnal seizures may present as urinary incontinence. Precipitants are occasionally identifiable if seizures are repeated. The duration of the seizure and postictal drowsiness and the presence of transient neurological symptoms may be of prognostic value. Additional symptoms to be specifically elicited would be headache, visual disturbance and vomiting, all indicating the possibility of raised intracranial pressure.

In the past history pay special attention to perinatal events, development and immunisation history. Serious illnesses and hospitalisation may be relevant. School attainments may be of diagnostic (petit mal) and prognostic value. A family history should be elicited. Try to be specific – 'epilepsy' may indicate post-traumatic seizures or tuberous sclerosis! The social background is relevant in making treatment decisions.

Many conditions may mimic epileptiform seizures. The commonest are listed in Table 29.1.

- Reflex anoxic events are profound vasovagal attacks. In response to stimuli such as pain, the child has a brief period of asystole evidenced by pallor and loss of consciousness. Recovery is usually instantaneous though occasionally some clonic jerking occurs. These events are particularly common in early infancy.
- Benign neonatal sleep myoclonus commonly occurs in the first month. Repetitive clonic jerking mainly of the upper limbs is noted during sleep. The movements cease when the child is woken. Examination and investigations are normal and the episodes subside usually by 4 months of age.
- Jitteriness/myoclonus is a normal phenomenon in the neonate. Movements can be abolished if the affected limb is firmly held.
- Cyanotic attacks are ill defined episodes typically occurring in the neonatal period. The infant may appear to gag or choke, become cyanosed and then gradually recovers. These are especially common in the first 2–3 days. Consciousness is retained and the child is well immediately afterwards.
- Drug reactions are occasionally seen. Dramatic oculogyric phenomena may be encountered if antiemetics are used. The

Table 29.1 Causes of 'funny turns'

Reflex anoxic events
Benign sleep myoclonus
Jitteriness
Cyanotic episodes
Apparent life threatening events
Drug reactions
Breathholding attacks
Tics
Apnoea
Syncope
Masturbation
Tetany

symptoms may be reversed by diazepam or benztropine, or diphenhydramine.

- ALTE (apparent life threatening event). This was previously known as 'near miss cot death'. The infant is found apparently lifeless and requires artificial respiration and occasionally cardiac massage prior to recovery. Some treat the entity sceptically ('near myth cot death'), since the parents are unlikely to be calm, objective and detached observers. The risk of subsequent SIDS is, however, increased to approximately 1 in 60. Investigations to exclude sepsis and airway problems are indicated.
- Tics are involuntary repetitive movements, commonly involving facial muscles. Consciousness is retained and they may be voluntarily suppressed. The prognosis is good.
- Tetany may be due to hypocalcaemia or alkalosis (often due to hyperventilation). The characteristic posture is of carpopedal spasm, which is often painful.
- Breathholding attacks can occur in early infancy, but more typically involve the assertive toddler. Often in response to frustration, the child holds the breath in inspiration, becoming cyanosed with loss of consciousness. Recovery ensues following loss of voluntary control of respiration, though occasionally clonic jerking may occur. The episodes may be reinforced by parents who accede to the child's demands rather than risk a recurrence.
- Syncope typically affects older children and adolescents. A variety of stimuli such as pain, prolonged fasting or standing provoke increased vagal tone with bradycardia, pallor and hypotension culminating in loss of consciousness. Recovery is immediate when the patient is allowed to remain horizontal.
- Apnoea/periodic respirations are a normal pattern of breathing in some infants, especially the preterm. This pattern may be exaggerated to frank apnoea in the presence of intercurrent respiratory infections. Apnoea is usually passive, the child being hypotonic and lifeless. Apnoeic seizures are associated with a tonic posture often with an ensuing clonic phase.
- Masturbatory movement is common in toddlers. The repetitive motions and occasionally vacant stare may cause confusion, but a careful description of the events will usually allow accurate diagnosis.

Clinical examination

This is often uninformative but a thorough examination, if normal, will reassure the family and physician. Of particular importance are weight (calculation of drug dosage) and head circumference. Hypertension may rarely present with seizures. Skin manifestations of neurocutaneous syndromes may be evident. Neurological examination will help exclude signs of tumour or degenerative illness. Inducing hyperventilation may precipitate petit mal absences or tetany, allowing clear diagnosis.

Investigation

The diagnosis of a seizure disorder is largely clinical; additional investigations are confirmatory or to assist prognosis. The EEG is the most frequently requested. This may show spikes in 2 per cent of normal children and is often normal in established epilepsy. Provocative manoeuvres such as photic stimulation or sleep deprivation and sleeping EEG may increase the yield. A specific EEG diagnosis may be made, e.g. petit mal, focal epilepsy, infantile spasms. Biochemical investigations are sometimes indicated if atypical features suggest tetany or inborn metabolic problems. CT or MRI scan is indicated if a tumour is suspected, though isolated epilepsy is a rare presentation of a space-occupying lesion. Opinions vary considerably regarding the indications for CT – features of raised intracranial pressure, focal seizures in early childhood or unusually refractory seizures are some of the more commonly agreed indications. Where possible a specific diagnosis of seizure type should be reached, bearing in mind the age and the description of the seizure, to allow more rational decision-making regarding management.

Education

Community perception of seizures and epilepsy is negative. The family should be given a clear explanation of the problem, its natural history and the therapeutic options. Parents may react to the diagnosis with a modified grief response – this should be acknowledged and sympathetic support provided. For patients, particularly older children, 'loss of control' and social embarrassment are the main worries. A generally optimistic tone is appropriate, given the favourable prognosis and response to treatment in most cases.

Practical advice on the management of a seizure is valuable – lay the patient semiprone, do not put anything in the mouth, use rectal diazepam if prolonged. Whilst seizure control is established, some restrictions on activity are appropriate – no swimming alone, no cycling in traffic and no bathing with the bathroom door locked. The legal implications of seizures should be clear. Patients with no daytime seizures for 2 years may apply for a driving licence.

Therapeutic options should be openly discussed. In some instances prophylaxis is unnecessary. In marginal cases, social factors and parental attitudes will be important in deciding on a therapeutic plan. Compliance with treatment is more likely when the family understand and agree with the treatment.

Drug treatment

'Primum non nocere' (first do no harm). In many cases anticonvulsant prophylaxis is inappropriate – a single seizure, a simple febrile convulsion and some cases of benign focal epilepsy, for example. Intermittent treatment with rectal diazepam may be a more effective strategy in some instances. Where regular prophylaxis is started, single drug treatment (monotherapy) is best. If the response to one drug is unsatisfactory, switch to another agent. Combinations of drugs sometimes reduce seizure frequency, but are more likely to increase side effects. Regular supervision is necessary to ensure good seizure control, compliance with treatment and avoidance of side effects. Monitoring of blood levels of anticonvulsants has a role, though its limitations should be recognised. The 'therapeutic range' is more a 'target' range. Good seizure control is possible with 'low' levels and enhanced seizure control with no side effects may be obtained in the 'toxic' range.

The aim of management should be to achieve as normal a lifestyle as possible. In some instances complete abolition of seizures may be impossible or achieved only at the expense of severe side effects. It is important to accept therapeutic failure when it occurs and to ensure that drug side effects are not added to the patient's problems.

Key points

- Funny turns are more common than seizures.
- Pallid attacks are more common in infancy.
- A clear description of events is the most important diagnostic item.
- Anticonvulsant treatment is not generally indicated after a single seizure.

Useful literature

- *The epilepsies of childhood*, N. O'Donohoe (Butterworth, 1985)

30 Headache

Headache is a common symptom affecting as many as one in five schoolchildren each year. Headaches can be divided into acute (of a few hours duration) or recurrent (months or years). Both types cause great parental fear of serious conditions. Parents fear meningitis in acute onset headache although viral infection is the commonest cause. Recurrent headache raises fears of a brain tumour although in the vast majority of cases no cause is found. A systematic approach is important both to reassure parents and to avoid diagnostic error.

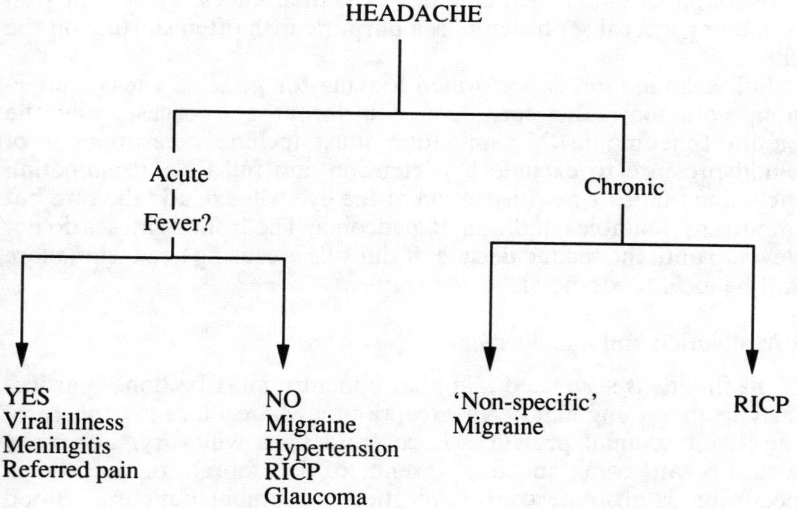

Fig. 30.1 Diagnostic pathway for headache

Acute headache

History

Document the site, severity, character and radiation of the pain. Note preceding or accompanying symptoms and any aggravating or relieving factors. Ask specifically for any symptoms suggestive of infection (e.g. fever or rash) or raised intracranial pressure (i.e. vomiting, drowsiness or visual disturbance). Recent drug ingestion may be relevant, e.g. indomethacin may cause headache. Elicit symptoms that might suggest a site of referred pain, for example pleuritic pain, dysphagia or otalgia.

Examination

The presence or absence of pyrexia should be noted. If the child is pyrexial it is important to note and record any signs of meningism. The examination note should state whether the child looked well or ill, had any neck stiffness or rash. Neck stiffness is best elicited, particularly in the younger child, by watching neck movements as the child follows a teddy bear or toy. Any screaming pyrexial toddler will have some degree of neck resistance rather than stiffness when their head is lifted without warning from the bed. Older children can be asked to hold a piece of paper under their chin or to kiss their knees. The classic rash of meningococcal septicaemia is a purpuric rash often starting on the chest.

Full examination is performed looking for possible sites of infection, commonly the ear, nose and throat and occasionally the pleura (pneumonia). Examination must include measurement of blood pressure to exclude hypertension and full CNS examination including fundoscopy. Inspection of the eye will exclude the rare but important treatable condition of glaucoma. The frontal sinuses do not develop until the second decade; if sinusitis is causing headache, there will be local tenderness.

Investigation and management

If meningitis is suspected a lumbar puncture must be done, particularly in the young child. An exception is where there is concern of raised intracranial pressure. Local guidelines will vary, but many would regard coma and the presence of decerebrate or decorticate posturing as absolute contraindications to lumbar puncture. Blood culture is usually positive since meningitis is invariably preceded by septicaemia. The urine can be checked for antigens and if clinically necessary, a lumbar puncture can be performed later. Viral infections require only simple analgesia. Specific problems, for example acute hypertension, require specific treatment.

Recurrent headache

History

The history is crucial in discriminating between the two common causes of headache, non-specific and migraine, and in excluding the uncommon but important headache associated with a brain tumour. As with acute headaches a full description of the attacks must be taken, asking the child what he experiences. This may be at variance with the parents' story. Ask the parents whether the child looks unwell or has to stop what he is doing. It is important to establish whether the child is well between these attacks of headache and whether there are any associated features. These would include anorexia, clumsiness, decrease in school performance, head tilt, tiredness and weight loss. Head tilt and headache point to posterior fossa pathology. Past medical history and all medications must be noted. A full social and family history must include questions about the family composition, family history of migraine or headaches and schooling.

The commonest diagnosis is non-specific headache. The child will often vividly describe the type of headache but paradoxically will find it difficult to give an exact description of its site. Words such as 'everywhere' and 'all over' are commonly used. The attacks are characteristically constant, daily and present for long periods of time. Despite this dramatic history the patient is able to play games and watch television although school days may be lost. The child complains of headache but looks well. Although nausea is common, vomiting is rare. There is often associated abdominal pain or other pains but never neurological complications such as hemiplegia. Establish when these headaches occur. 'Headaches of convenience' are not just marital, but may be helpful in avoiding school subjects that the child does not like, for example, mathematics.

The important differential is migraine. Migrainous headaches are often throbbing and, unlike non-specific headaches, will be localised to an area. This may be bifrontal or occipital rather than unilateral. It is important to ask about any prodromal symptoms. Some children can draw a visual scotoma better than describe one. A crucial distinction is that in migraine there will be a history of attacks lasting hours or days, but between these episodes the child will be completely normal. This cannot be overemphasised. The younger child may be unable to articulate his pain or may begin with attacks of abdominal pain associated with vomiting. As the child gets older the more classic attacks of an aura or often just a period of irritability followed by a severe throbbing unilateral headache associated with nausea and vomiting will occur. Although nausea may occur in non-specific headaches vomiting will occur in migraine.

Unlike non-specific headaches, children with migraine prefer to lie down in a quiet dark place and sleep until the attack has passed. There is a family history of migraine in over 90 per cent of children and indeed the diagnosis must be viewed with suspicion where this is absent. It must be remembered that migraine may be complicated and associated with transient hemiparesis or occasionally ophthalmoplegia.

The headaches of intracranial tumours are often occipital, but may be frontal if the tumour is supratentorial. It is essential to remember the classic description of the headache of raised intracranial pressure. This headache begins early in the morning and is associated with, and eased by, effortless vomiting. Children prefer to stay still and not cry out and initially it may be mistaken for school avoidance. As the intracranial pressure increases, unsteadiness is usually noted and drowsiness will occur. Although parents become more concerned when headaches last over a year, the headaches of intracranial tumour are likely to be of only a few months duration and usually associated with other symptoms and signs.

It is important to remember that the symptoms of raised intracranial pressure can also be due to hydrocephalus or benign raised intracranial pressure. The salient point of history in benign raised intracranial pressure is that it often occurs following otitis media or withdrawal of steroids. Other causes include oral contraceptives as well as the antibiotics tetracycline and nalidixic acid though many cases are idiopathic. Many children are relatively asymptomatic for long periods, but may then present with double vision secondary to a sixth nerve palsy. Diagnosis is by exclusion when the CT scan shows no evidence of hydrocephalus or tumour.

Two other conditions are worth noting. Remember headache may be the first sign of meningeal leukaemia. Secondly patients with cyanotic heart disease who present with prominent headache must be suspected of having a brain abscess until proven otherwise.

Examination

It is imperative to record the child's head circumference. The head circumference that is out of proportion to the child's weight should arouse suspicion. A cracked pot note over the coronal sutures when tapping is a valuable sign of raised intracranial pressure. Cardiovascular examination must include measuring the blood pressure and listening for carotid and cranial bruits. Severe hypertension is an important treatable cause of headache.

Full neurological examination is mandatory. The child's gait should be noted, looking for ataxia. The cranial nerves should be examined fully and the fundi checked for papilloedema. It should be remembered, however, that significant intracranial pressure may exist without papilloedema and its absence does not exclude it. The formal neurological examination should look for any asymmetrical signs or the presence of hyperreflexia with upgoing plantars in the lower limbs, consistent with raised intracranial pressure. It is important to form an impression of the child's mental state, whether they are tense or depressed and the parents' reaction to the history and examination. A full physical examination includes the ear, nose, throat, the chest and sinuses to exclude any referred pain.

Investigation and management

The majority of children with recurrent headache have non-specific pain and the most important investigation is time. It is important to take a thorough history and examination as above. If the history is of non-specific headache and examination is normal then it can be emphasised to the child and the parents that nothing serious can be found. Parental concerns about serious pathologies such as cerebral tumour should be brought out in the open. There are no diagnostic tests for non-specific headaches or indeed migraine and these diagnoses must be made on the history and full clinical examination. It is often important to see the child again in a few weeks and again ask for any new symptoms and fully examine the child. This use of time is a better investigation than an automatic referral for CT scan.

Where migraine is diagnosed a search for dietary precipitants is occasionally rewarding – chocolate, citrus fruits and cheese may be implicated. Symptomatic analgesia and antiemetic treatments are effective in the majority. Where attacks are severe, ergotamine may be used. If attacks are frequent, propranolol may be used as prophylaxis.

Clearly if a child does have symptoms or signs of raised intracranial pressure they need an urgent CT scan and neurosurgical opinion.

Although an important group in headaches, they are the exception rather than the rule.

Key points

- Most children with headaches have common non-serious conditions. Proper history combined with examination will help differentiate the serious conditions.
- Headache is common in children.
- The family history is usually positive in migraine.
- Isolated headache is rarely due to tumour.
- Early morning headache, vomiting without nausea and visual disturbance suggest raised intracranial pressure.
- Time and reassurance are often the most helpful treatments.

Useful literature

- *Migraine in childhood*, J. Hockaday (Butterworth, 1988)

31 Murmur

Introduction

A murmur is audible turbulent blood flow within the heart or great vessels. If the turbulence is created by a structural abnormality, the murmur is organic. If, however, the turbulence occurs in a structurally normal heart, the murmur is innocent or benign. One per cent of all children born have a structural heart defect and most of these have an organic murmur, while 40–50 per cent of healthy school children have innocent murmurs.

Despite the value of a murmur as a clinical sign, it is essential that it is not considered to be the beginning and the end of the cardiovascular examination. While a murmur may facilitate the clinical diagnosis of the anatomical cardiac defect, it gives little information about the functional significance of such a lesion. It should also be remembered that serious congenital and acquired heart disease may be present without a murmur, for example, in transposition of the great arteries and myocarditis respectively.

Equally, it is important that we do not create heart disease where none exists, e.g. the child with the innocent murmur, and should not overlook a significant though sometimes subtle structural defect, e.g. a coarctation of the aorta or an atrial septal defect.

The primary responsibility of the general practitioner or paediatrician, therefore, is to try and separate those children who have normal cardiac function and normal cardiac anatomy with an innocent murmur from those who have disturbed cardiac function, abnormal cardiac anatomy and an organic murmur. The latter require referral to a paediatric cardiologist for more detailed evaluation.

History

A careful and detailed history should be ascertained. The age and the circumstances in which the murmur was first noted may give useful clues. Murmurs first noted during a febrile illness are commonly innocent. Enquire as to the presence of cardiac symptoms such as breathlessness, cyanosis or palpitations. In the past history document any medications taken, or any serious illness during pregnancy. A family history of congenital heart disease should be sought.

Examination

A full clinical examination should be carried out. Growth should be measured and plotted on appropriate centile charts. Look specifically for any dysmorphic features which would suggest any of the syndromes with cardiac problems, e.g. Down's syndrome, Williams' syndrome, Turner syndrome or Noonan's syndrome. The presence of clubbing should suggest the possibility of cyanotic congenital heart disease.

Palpate the peripheral pulses and ensure that there is no brachiofemoral delay. Accurate measurement of the blood pressure in the upper limb should be part of routine assessment and measurement of lower limb blood pressure is indicated if there is any suspicion of coarctation of the aorta. Inspect the praecordium for any evidence of chest deformity. Localise the position and character of the apex beat and palpate also for any impulses, sounds and thrills, paying particular attention to the suprasternal notch and the supraclavicular areas.

Auscultation should then begin with an assessment of the heart sounds, using first the bell and then the diaphragm of the stethoscope. The first heart sound should be auscultated at the apex and the lower left sternal border and the second heart sound at the aortic and pulmonary areas. The sounds should be assessed for intensity – normal, increased or decreased and for evidence of splitting. The first sound is commonly split and splitting of the second sound, which should vary with respiration, is expected in all healthy children. Evaluation of the pulmonary component of the second heart sound is one of the most important auscultatory skills in clinical cardiology. A normal P2 indicates normal pulmonary arterial pressure. An increased P2 suggests pulmonary hypertension, while a decreased intensity indicates that pulmonary pressure is low, as occurs in moderate or severe pulmonary stenosis.

Physiological splitting occurs in normal healthy children and in those with minor congenital abnormalities, such as a small ventricular defect. Exaggerated splitting occurs with pulmonary valve stenosis, while fixed splitting is a cardinal sign of an atrial septal defect. Fixed splitting implies that there is less than a 20 millisecond variation in split during the respiratory cycle. The normal heart sounds are heard well with both the bell and the diaphragm, though in small infants the splitting of the second heart sound may be more clearly appreciated with the diaphragm. Additional sounds such as a third heart sound and fourth heart sound, which are low pitched, may be heard only with the bell and ejection clicks which are high frequency sounds may be appreciated only with the diaphragm.

When assessing murmurs, a similar methodical approach should apply. Murmurs should be listened to with both the bell and the diaphragm of the stethoscope. They should be assessed for:

1. timing, i.e. systolic, diastolic or continuous,
2. frequency,
3. intensity,
4. site of maximum intensity,
5. radiation,
6. quality and in some cases,
7. variation with posture,
8. variation with respiration,
9. response to exercise, and
10. response to the Valsalva manoeuvre.

Timing

Systolic murmurs may occur in early to midsystole and murmurs in this part of systole are commonly ejection or crescendo/decrescendo in type and most are related to turbulent blood flow within the left or right ventricular outflow tract. In the structurally normal heart, the majority of the stroke volume is ejected in the first half of systole and therefore innocent ejection systolic murmurs are confined to this portion of the cardiac cycle and are never pansystolic. If, on the other hand, there is obstruction at pulmonary or aortic valve level, then ejection is prolonged and the duration of the murmur lengthened. The peak of the crescendo murmur, therefore, varies with the severity of the outflow obstruction, so that in mild pulmonary stenosis, the murmur peaks in the first half of systole and as the obstruction becomes more severe, the peak occurs later in systole and the murmur becomes longer in duration.

This situation exists when all of the blood in the right ventricle has to be ejected through the right ventricular outflow tract. If, however, there is an associated ventricular septal defect, such as in the tetralogy of Fallot, some of the blood can be diverted through the ventricular septal defect into the aorta. When the outflow tract obstruction becomes more severe in this setting, the murmur becomes shorter and softer as less blood traverses the narrowed infundibular area, creating less turbulence. In the child with tetralogy, this is an important sign of increasing outflow obstruction. In the presence of a hypercyanotic spell, the murmur may disappear altogether. With aortic valve stenosis, the behaviour of the murmur is similar to that in isolated pulmonary valve stenosis.

The classic late systolic murmur or honk, due to mitral valve prolapse, is usually heard at the apex and follows a midsystolic click. The murmur is related to a mild degree of mitral regurgitation.

Pansystolic murmurs are usually plateau in nature and suggest either mitral regurgitation, tricuspid regurgitation or a ventricular septal defect. While the classic description of a murmur associated with a ventricular septal defect is that of a plateau pansystolic murmur, this is not always the case and it depends on the size of the defect, the pulmonary vascular resistance and the position of the communication within the ventricular septum. At both ends of the spectrum, in the presence of normal pulmonary vascular resistance, the murmur may be soft and early to midsystolic. In the case of a very small muscular lesion, for example, the murmur may be decrescendo, as the defect becomes obliterated because of active septal muscular contraction during systole. With large defects, on the other hand, there may be insufficient restriction to create pansystolic turbulence. Of course, as pulmonary vascular resistance increases, the duration of the murmur in large defects also becomes shortened and ultimately disappears as pulmonary vascular resistance equals or supersedes systemic, as in the Eisenmenger syndrome.

Diastolic murmurs also need to be auscultated with the bell and the diaphragm and they may be early, mid, late (presystolic) or indeed pandiastolic in duration. Diastolic murmurs are never innocent. Early decrescendo diastolic murmurs are usually due to semilunar valve incompetence. The most common mid-diastolic murmurs in congenital heart disease are caused by turbulent blood flow across the mitral valve and tricuspid valves in the presence of large left to right shunts at ventricular and atrial level respectively. The late diastolic murmur or presystolic murmur is associated with organic mitral stenosis and was commonly heard when rheumatic heart disease was prevalent.

A continuous murmur by definition is one which starts in systole and extends in an unbroken manner through the second heart sound into diastole. It may extend throughout both systole and diastole, but this is not always the case. The classic continuous murmur is due to a patent ductus arteriosus and the duration of the murmur as well as the intensity will vary depending on the size of the ductus and the pulmonary vascular resistance. Other causes of a continuous murmur include an aortopulmonary window, systemic to pulmonary artery shunts, coronary fistulae and systemic arteriovenous fistulae, e.g. hepatic, pulmonary, cerebral.

The most common continuous murmur, however, is the benign venous hum, related to turbulent blood flow in the systemic veins of the neck. While the organic murmurs have systolic accentuation, the venous hum has diastolic accentuation.

The continuous murmur should be distinguished from a to and fro murmur, a term which implies a separate systolic ejection murmur and decrescendo diastolic murmur, such as would be heard with aortic stenosis and aortic incompetence.

Frequency

Frequency or pitch refers to the number of cycles per second or hertz, which are present in the murmur. Murmurs may be of low, medium or high frequency. Examples of low frequency murmurs would include diastolic rumbles or the innocent systolic ejection murmur, and these are best heard with the bell of the stethoscope. Highpitched murmurs, on the other hand, such as the decrescendo diastolic murmur of aortic regurgitation, may be heard only with the diaphragm. The pansystolic murmur of the ventricular septal defect and the continuous murmur of the ductus arteriosus are medium to highpitched.

It is important to use both the bell and the diaphragm of the stethoscope as the pitch of the murmur may help in differentiating the cause of a particular murmur, e.g. an early decrescendo diastolic murmur heard at the upper left sternal border, if best heard with the bell, suggests a pulmonary aetiology whereas if heard only with the diaphragm, this is almost always due to aortic regurgitation unless the pulmonary regurgitant murmur is associated with severe pulmonary hypertension.

Intensity

The intensity or loudness of a murmur is measured in decibels and is assessed clinically using a grading system of 1 to 6, as outlined by Zuberbuhler. Grade I implies a murmur that is barely audible and may not be immediately apparent on initial auscultation. Grade II is soft, but immediately heard. Grade III is a loud murmur but without an associated thrill. When a thrill is present, the murmur is grade IV or louder. A grade V murmur can be heard with just the edge of the tilted stethoscope head in contact with the skin and the grade VI murmur can be heard with a stethoscope removed from the chest wall.

The intensity of a murmur should not be used in isolation as an indication of severity. While it is true that in the presence of aortic stenosis, the louder the murmur, in general the more severe the obstruction, this is not always the case and in the small infant with critical aortic stenosis, the murmur may, in fact, be very soft or even absent. The correlation between intensity of the murmur and the size of a ventricular septal defect or patent ductus arteriosus is even less reliable so that you may have a loud murmur with an associated thrill with a small or moderate to large defect. On the other hand, with a very large defect or indeed with a very small defect, the murmur may be no more than grade II in intensity.

Site of maximum intensity

The site of maximum intensity of a murmur may help to establish the underlying anatomical defect. For example, a pansystolic murmur which is heard maximally at the fourth left intercostal space at the left sternal border is likely to be a ventricular septal defect, whereas a pansystolic murmur heard maximally at the apex would favour mitral regurgitation. Similarly, an ejection systolic murmur that is maximally heard in the second right intercostal space would favour a left ventricular outflow tract obstructive lesion, while if a similar murmur was heard in the second left intercostal space, it would suggest a pulmonary valve lesion.

Radiation

An appreciation of the radiation of the murmur will complement the findings outlined above and may consolidate the clinical diagnosis of the underlying cardiac defect. For example, a pansystolic murmur at the apex which radiates to the axilla is likely to be due to mitral regurgitation, while an ejection systolic murmur over the base of the heart with radiation to the axilla and lungs suggests a pulmonary valvular and/or pulmonary branch origin for the turbulent blood flow. An ejection systolic murmur due to aortic stenosis radiates to the carotid arteries.

Quality

This is a purely descriptive term, but again may be helpful in clarifying the diagnosis, e.g. the pansystolic ventricular septal defect murmur is often rough in quality while that due to mitral regurgitation is smoother and more blowing in quality. The innocent ejection systolic murmur of Still, often described as musical, has a pure tone that is due to regular frequency characteristics. Some terms used may be unhelpful such as the description of the continuous murmur due to a ductus arteriosus as being machinery in type. This infers a roughness and loudness to the murmur which is often not present and, if expected, may confuse rather than facilitate the diagnosis. The quality of the murmur should be described as it sounds to the examiner rather than by any traditional term.

Variation with posture

It is often important to examine a patient in both the supine and erect posture as this may alter the haemodynamics and in so doing, change the character and intensity of a murmur. The innocent venous hum, for example, is heard with the patient in the sitting position but is abolished by laying the patient supine, as this eliminates the hydrostatic gradient which creates the turbulent blood flow in the major veins entering the right heart. The innocent precordial ejection murmur of Still, on the other hand, is maximally heard in the supine position and often diminishes or indeed disappears with the patient standing. The left ventricular outflow ejection murmur found in patients with hypertrophic obstructive cardiomyopathy conversely may increase in intensity in the standing position, due to a decrease in the left ventricular end diastolic volume, thus narrowing the left ventricular outlet, and diminish in intensity in the supine posture with an increase in left ventricular end diastolic volume. These changes in volume also influence the behaviour of the murmur and click in association with mitral valve prolapse. With the maximum end diastolic volume in the supine position, the mitral valve leaflets may be adequately accommodated to the cavity of the left ventricle and oppose one another without evidence of mitral regurgitation. A click often heard in midsystole is a clinical marker for mitral prolapse in the supine position. In the standing position, with a drop in left ventricular end diastolic volume, the click moves earlier in systole and the valve leaflets prolapse further into the left atrium and may become incompetent, giving rise to the late systolic murmur classically heard in this condition. Squatting, by increasing left ventricular end diastolic volume, will also diminish the signs of prolapse as well as reducing the left ventricular outflow tract turbulence in the presence of obstructive cardiomyopathy.

Proper positioning of the patient may be essential if important diagnoses are not to be overlooked. For example, in the presence of mild aortic regurgitation, the soft highpitched decrescendo diastolic murmur may only be heard with the patient sitting up, leaning forward and with breath held in expiration. Similarly, diastolic rumbles, related to inflow turbulence across the mitral valve, may only be heard with the patient in the left lateral decubitus position and auscultating over the apex.

Variation with respiration

Murmurs generated by turbulent blood flow in the right heart tend to be exaggerated by inspiration, which increases the venous return to the heart.

Variation, if any, should be assessed initially during normal quiet respiration. The murmur of tricuspid regurgitation in particular increases with inspiration, so that a pansystolic or even midsystolic plateau murmur heard at the mid or lower left sternal border, which increases during inspiration, suggests tricuspid regurgitation rather than a ventricular septal defect. Also the diastolic rumble, created by turbulent blood flow across the tricuspid valve in the presence of an atrial septal defect, may increase during the inspiratory phase of respiration.

Response to exercise

Where there is uncertainty about the significance of a murmur under resting conditions, exercise may help to clarify the issue. With an increase in cardiac output, all murmurs tend to become more prominent. However, the quality, the duration and the radiation may help to decide whether the murmur is innocent or organic. More importantly, exercise may exaggerate or produce additional heart sounds, especially ejection clicks which will identify a semilunar valve abnormality and establish an organic cause for the turbulent blood flow. While the lesion may not be functionally important, the patient may require antibiotic prophylaxis for dental therapy, e.g. bicuspid aortic valve.

Valsalva manoeuvre

The physiological and haemodynamic changes during this manoeuvre are complex. However, the innocent murmur tends to diminish or disappear during it while the murmur associated with hypertrophic obstructive cardiomyopathy may increase in intensity due to a decrease in left ventricular end diastolic volume.

Table 31.1 summarises some of the more common findings which may help to differentiate an innocent from an organic murmur.

Investigations

It is often possible on the basis of a careful history and complete cardiovascular evaluation to arrive at an accurate clinical diagnosis, though this may not be the case in the sick neonate. The vast majority of children with innocent murmurs do not require additional tests or

Table 31.1 Clinical features which help differentiate innocent from organic murmurs

Innocent	*Organic*
	Cardiac symptoms
Normal pulses	Abnormal pulses
Normal apical position and activity	Displaced apex
Normal precordial activity	1 LV activity
	1 RV activity
	Thrill
Normal heart sounds	Abnormal heart sounds
Systolic murmur < Gr II/VI	Murmur ≥ Gr III/IV
Early ejection systolic murmur	Pansystolic
	Diastolic
Low frequency	Medium to high frequency
Well localised	Wide radiation
Variation with posture	Radiation to axillae or neck

The above lists outline some findings which favour an innocent versus an organic murmur and vice versa. Those outlined favouring an innocent murmur do not exclude an organic lesion, which may not have functional significance, such as a small ventricular septal defect.

investigations. If there is doubt, however, or if the history or physical examination suggests an organic lesion, then additional investigations are indicated and the infant or child should be evaluated by a paediatric cardiologist.

The standard investigations include the chest X-ray, and electrocardiogram. The chest X-ray gives information on cardiac size and shape, as well as perhaps chamber enlargement, and an evaluation of pulmonary vasculature, while the electrocardiogram is used to evaluate hypertrophy of the atria or ventricles, as well as any abnormality of cardiac rhythm. It is important to remember, however, that you can have a normal chest X-ray and electrocardiogram in the presence of significant cardiac disease, for example in aortic stenosis. In the newborn infant, it can be especially difficult to arrive at an accurate anatomical diagnosis on the basis of clinical examination, even with a chest X-ray and electrocardiogram. In 25 per cent of cases, the diagnosis is inaccurate. With the advent of echocardiography and the more recent addition of Doppler interrogation of blood flow within the heart, the non-invasive assessment of congenital heart disease is both highly sensitive and specific in 98 per cent of cases. In older infants and children, clinical examination is highly accurate and the non-invasive tests are used to arrive at a complete evaluation of the functional significance of the underlying cardiac defect.

Cardiac catheterisation remains the gold standard. However, it is a procedure that is used less and less for diagnostic purposes with the advent of echo Doppler studies and is increasingly used during interventional procedures to treat specific heart defects, for example, balloon pulmonary valvuloplasty for pulmonary valve stenosis.

Education

Since the vast majority of children who have murmurs will have normal hearts, it is important that if a murmur is considered to be innocent, the parents are reassured to this effect and the child is not brought back for unnecessary review. It is often reassuring for parents to be told that the murmur that their child has is a sign of a healthy heart and circulation. No precautions of any sort are required and, of course, antibiotic prophylaxis with dental therapy is unnecessary.

The majority of children with congenital heart defects, whether they have required surgery or not, can lead an unrestricted life and can participate in school and normal childhood activities. Restriction in terms of competitive sport is limited to a small number of patients who may be at an increased risk of sudden death, for example, those with hypertrophic cardiomyopathy, severe aortic stenosis and selected patients following repair of tetralogy of Fallot, transposition of the great arteries and tricuspid atresia.

It is often difficult for parents to give the children the freedom they need to develop as individuals if they have been chronically sick prior to their corrective cardiac surgery. It is important however for the psychological health of the children that this transition does occur and this should be facilitated by the supportive role of the medical staff involved in the child's care.

Key points

- Innocent murmurs can be detected in up to 50 per cent of healthy children.
- Listen carefully – especially to the heart sounds.
- The main decision is – innocent or organic?
- Echocardiography is the most valuable investigation.

Useful literature

- *Understanding paediatric heart sounds*, S. Lehrer (W.B. Saunders, 1992)
- *Clinical diagnosis in paediatric cardiology*, J. Zuberbuhler (Churchill Livingstone, 1981)

32 Neonatal cholestasis

Introduction

Jaundice in the neonatal period occurs in up to 60 per cent of term and 80 per cent of preterm babies. Typically the increased serum bilirubin is unconjugated, occurring on day 2 to 3 of life in a well baby who is tolerating feeds. In the majority of these infants, jaundice resolves spontaneously. Pathological jaundice is likely in the following circumstances:

- jaundice in the first 24 hours of life – haemolysis;
- jaundiced and unwell – sepsis, metabolic;
- persistent jaundice after 10 days or conjugated hyperbilirubinaemiac (direct bilirubin > 25mmol).

This chapter will focus on the latter (Fig. 32.1).

The immediate aim of investigating infants with cholestasis is to detect the following:

1. extrahepatic biliary atresia for which surgery is imperative under 50 days of age;
2. inherited metabolic conditions which could be life-threatening;
3. other treatable conditions, e.g. sepsis.

Causes of prolonged hyperbilirubinaemia are categorised according to whether the jaundice is primarily unconjugated or conjugated (Table 32.1). In approximately 50 per cent of neonates with conjugated hyperbilirubinaemia, investigations will reveal an underlying diagnosis of extra-hepatic biliary atresia or α1-antitrypsin deficiency. The remainder are mainly children with non-specific liver disease for which the term 'neonatal hepatitis' is used. In the majority of these children the hepatitis ultimately resolves. However before a diagnosis

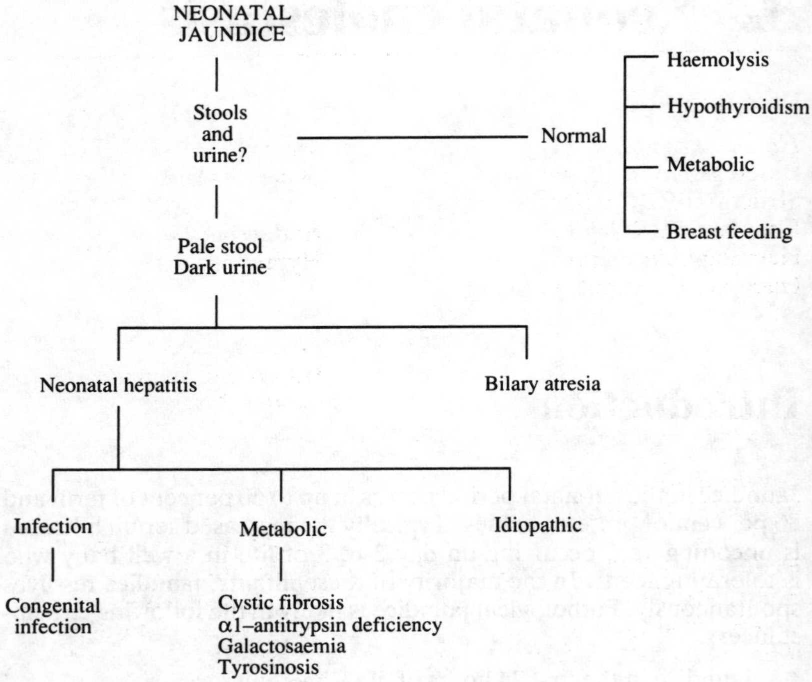

Fig. 32.1 Diagnostic pathway for neonatal jaundice

of 'idiopathic neonatal hepatitis' is made, all of the conditions outlined in Table 32.1 must be excluded. It is vitally important to diagnose biliary atresia before 6 weeks of age. The condition is associated with progressive inflammatory destruction of the biliary tree and is not an anatomical 'atresia' as the name suggests. Surgery undertaken before eight weeks of age will improve or clear jaundice in the majority. The results of surgery in older infants are very poor and transplantation may be the only option.

Assessment of a 'cholestatic' infant

Infants with cholestasis should be assessed in a standardised manner starting with a comprehensive history, followed by a careful clinical

Table 32.1 Causes of prolonged neonatal jaundice

Unconjugated	
Haematological	*Metabolic*
Blood group incompatibility	Galactosaemia
Structural RBC defect	
Enzymatic RBC defect	*Endocrine*
Haemoglobinopathy	Hypothyroidism
Haematoma, caput, bruising	
	Miscellaneous
	Breast milk jaundice
	Crigler–Najjar
Conjugated	
'Idiopathic' neonatal hepatitis	*Metabolic*
	Antitrypsin deficiency
Extrahepatic biliary obstruction	Cystic fibrosis
Biliary atresia	Galactosaemia
Choledochal cyst	Neonatal iron storage disease
Bile sludge (post TPN)	
	Fructose intolerance
	Tyrosinaemia
Intrahepatic	Gaucher's disease
Alagille's syndrome	Niemann–Pick's disease
Non-syndromic paucity of bile ducts	Wolman's disease
Byler's disease	
'Inspissated' bile syndrome (after severe haemolysis).	*Endocrine*
	Hypopituitarism
	Hypothyroidism
Infective	
Congenital infection (TORCH viruses)	
Hepatitis B and C	
Listeria	
Syphilis	
Sepsis / urinary tract infection	

examination before proceeding to laboratory investigations (Table 32.2).

History

Important clues regarding the type of jaundice can be obtained immediately on enquiring about the nature of stools and urine being passed by the baby. Green stools imply that the biliary tree is patent. Pale stools and dark urine are indicative of a biliary stasis due to hepatic injury or bile duct obstruction.

Enquiries should be made regarding consanguinity (inborn errors of metabolism) and the presence of flu-like symptoms or exposure to cats during pregnancy (toxoplasmosis, rubella, etc.). Document neonatal details including birthweight and head circumference of the infant (congenital infection), methods and type of feeding, periods of hypoglycaemia (inborn errors of metabolism, hypopituitarism) or purpuric skin rashes (congenital infection). The family history may reveal information regarding previously affected children with metabolic defects, intrahepatic cholestasis, α1-antitrypsin (A1AT) deficiency, hypothyroidism or cystic fibrosis.

Clinical evaluation

Careful clinical examination of the jaundiced neonate is often rewarding. It may provide clues to the aetiology of the underlying condition especially if there are dysmorphic features. Down's syndrome may be associated with infantile hepatitis. In Alagille's syndrome, a broad forehead, deep widely spaced eyes, a long straight nose, underdeveloped mandible and growth retardation may be seen, biliary hypoplasia causing the jaundice.

Eye

Examination should exclude the presence of cataracts (congenital infection, galactosaemia), posterior embryotoxin (Alagille's syndrome), choroidoretinitis (congenital infection, Zellweger's and Alagille's syndrome) and optic nerve hypoplasia (septo-optic dysplasia).

Skin

Widespread petechiae are suggestive of congenital infection and thrombocytopenia. Xanthomas, spider naevi and palmar erythema are rare in the neonatal period.

Cardiovascular system

Pulmonary branch stenosis occurs with Alagille's syndrome. Ventricular septal defects are found with increased frequency in Down's syndrome. Congenital heart disease is also associated with intrauterine infection.

Abdomen

In the neonatal period, the liver edge can be palpated 3 or 4 cm below the right subcostal border. By 4 months of age, this has decreased to 2 cm. Hepatosplenomegaly, if present, does not help in differentiating hepatocellular from obstructive causes of jaundice. It is important to document the consistency of the liver. A hard liver may suggest that fibrosis/cirrhosis are already present. A cystic mass below the liver should alert one to the possibility of a choledochal cyst.

Infants with prolonged jaundice and hypoglycaemia may have hypopituitarism. Penile hypoplasia in the male and midline clefts further suggest a pituitary problem.

Investigations

The initial aim is to differentiate conjugated from unconjugated hyperbilirubinaemia. In an outpatient clinic it is important to look for the presence of bilirubin or urobilinogen in the urine. The finding of bilirubin in the urine in large amounts implies conjugated hyperbilirubinaemia. In contrast, the presence of urobilinogen implies that there is biliary drainage into the intestine. Urinary findings are confirmed by checking serum levels of conjugated and unconjugated bilirubin.

No single laboratory test will completely distinguish intrahepatic from extrahepatic cholestasis. However, various combinations of tests may help identify specific causes of cholestasis and also assess the degree of hepatobiliary dysfunction (Table 32.2).

Hepatic enzymes

Elevated levels of aspartate aminotransferase (AST) and alanine

Table 32.2 Suggested work-up for cholestatic jaundice in the neonate

INITIAL TESTS	LATER TESTS
Blood	
FBC, reticulocyte count and Coombs	Early morning cortisol (if septo-optic dysplasia suspected)
SBR – direct and indirect	
AST/ALT/ gamma GT/Alk phos	
Albumin and PT ratio	Iron, ferritin
Cholesterol and triglycerides	Vitamins A, D and E
T4 and TSH	Copper/caeruloplasmin
α1-antitrypsin level and phenotype	Hepatitis A and C
Gal-1-phos uridyl transferase	
Amino acid screen	
TORCH and hepatitis B serology	
24° pre-meal sugar profile	
Urea and electrolytes, creatinine	
Ca/phosphate	
Urine	
Culture and sensitivity	Succinylacetone
Bilirubin/urobilinogen	
Reducing substances	
Amino acids	
CMV	
Radiology	
US of liver and spleen	Wrist
± HIDA	Vertebrae (?butterfly)
Ophthalmology	
Check for choroidoretinitis/post. embryotoxin/ cataract/cherry red spot	
Miscellaneous	
Immunoreactive trypsin	Bone marrow aspirate
Sweat test	Liver biopsy
	Skin biopsy

aminotransferase (ALT) are reflections of hepatocellular damage. Levels are increased to a greater extent in hepatitis than in extrahepatic biliary atresia.

Serum alkaline phosphatase is increased in conditions which interfere with bile excretion and therefore is increased in both hepatitis and bile duct obstruction. The enzyme is widely distributed throughout the body in liver, bone and intestine and is therefore not a specific marker for liver disease. However, alkaline phosphate isoenzymes can now be measured by electrophoresis to identify the source of increased levels.

Elevated levels of gamma glutamyl transferase (GGT) are almost always hepatic in origin and usually indicate cholestasis. A greater than fivefold elevation of GGT is supportive of a diagnosis of biliary atresia or α1–antitrypsin deficiency.

Serum proteins

Hypoalbuminaemia in association with chronic liver disease may be due to decreased synthesis, increased degradation of albumin and increased plasma volume. A low albumin is found most frequently in advanced liver disease and is therefore of limited diagnostic value in the neonatal period.

Clotting factors

Hepatocellular failure will ultimately result in abnormal clotting due to a decreased synthesis of all clotting factors except factor 8. The half life of these factors vary from a few hours to four days. Prothrombin time (PT) estimation is therefore an indirect, but simple method of assessing hepatic synthetic function.

α1-antitrypsin level

α1-antitrypsin deficiency is the most common diagnosis after extrahepatic biliary atresia in neonatal conjugated hyperbilirubinaemia. The diagnosis may be suspected on routine serum protein electrophoresis by finding a low or absent α1 globin fraction. Normal A1AT levels do not exclude a diagnosis of A1AT deficiency. A1AT is an acute phase reactant. Levels will increase in response to stresses, including infection. Therefore it is extremely important to document phenotype, as well as levels in suspected cases. Eight-five percent of the population have a PiMM phenotype with normal A1AT levels ranging between 200 and 400 mg/dl. Phenotypic variants associated with A1AT deficiency and liver disease are PiZZ (levels of between 20 and 160 mg/dl) and PiNULL (no A1AT activity).

Infection screen

Urine samples should be routinely checked for evidence of infection in any infant with prolonged jaundice. If the infant is clinically unwell and sepsis is suspected, a full septic work-up, including blood cultures and lumbar puncture, should be performed.

If congenital infection is suspected, TORCH titres (toxoplasmosis, rubella, cytomegalovirus, herpes simplex) from the infant should be compared against maternal titres. Blood should be reserved for VDRL in cases suspected of congenital syphilis. Urine from infants can be examined directly for cytomegalovirus (CMV). Hepatitis B is also a recognised cause of neonatal hepatitis, as is the human immunodeficiency virus (HIV).

Metabolic profile

The metabolic conditions found in association with conjugated hyperbilirubinaemia include galactosaemia, tyrosinaemia, hereditary fructose intolerance and neonatal iron storage disease (haemochromatosis). The latter three are extremely rare. The presence of reducing substances in the urine may provide clues to the diagnosis of galactosaemia or fructose intolerance. However, false negative results can be obtained if the baby is not receiving galactose containing food (galactosaemia), sucrose containing food (fructose intolerance) or is vomiting. Reducing substances can also appear in the urine in advanced liver disease due to other causes. Galactosaemia is diagnosed by measuring red blood cell galactose-1-phosphate uridyl transferase activity. Recent blood transfusions may invalidate the result. Tyrosinaemia may be screened for by testing for the presence of succinylacetone in the urine.

Metabolic screens (i.e. amino acid estimation) in the blood and urine are of limited value in liver disease. Elevated levels of amino acids including methionine and tyrosine may be due to severe liver disease and are not diagnostic of an underlying metabolic defect.

Sweat test

Cystic fibrosis can cause prolonged neonatal jaundice. In the neonatal period, raised plasma immunoreactive trypsin can be used as a screening procedure. The diagnosis must be confirmed with a sweat test after 4–6 weeks.

Endocrine

Hypothyroidism may present as prolonged jaundice. Classically this is an unconjugated hyperbilirubinaemia but hypothyroidism may also be associated with cholestasis. Cholestatic jaundice may accompany hypopituitarism and septo-optic dysplasia. This diagnosis is suspected if there is hypoglycaemia in the neonatal period and/or penile hypoplasia in males. Roving nystagmus may be seen secondary to optic nerve hypoplasia. Thyroxine and thyroid stimulating hormone (TSH), growth hormone, glucose levels and cortisol levels should be documented during hypoglycaemic episodes in an attempt to establish the diagnosis.

Radiological investigation

Ultrasound

Ultrasonography of liver and spleen, performed after 3–4 hours fasting, is an important adjunct to diagnosis in neonatal cholestasis. The absence of a gallbladder is suggestive but not diagnostic of extrahepatic biliary atresia. Cranial ultrasound may identify areas of calcification (intrauterine infection) or confirm absence of septum pellucidum in septo-optic dysplasia.

Radionucleoside imaging

Hepatobiliary scintigraphy, using technetium-labelled iminodiacetic acid analogues (IDA), may help differentiate biliary atresia from non-obstructive causes of cholestasis. IDA is taken up by the liver, concentrated by the biliary system and then excreted into the bowel. In extrahepatic biliary atresia with normal parenchymal function, uptake and concentration of the dye in the liver is normal. However, there is no excretion into the bowel. In neonatal hepatitis there is impaired uptake and concentration. There may also be delayed excretion into the bowel. The administration of phenobarbitone orally (5 mg/kg/day) for three days prior to this test maximises biliary excretion and increases the sensitivity of the test.

Liver biopsy

Liver biopsy remains the most reliable method of assessing liver pathology in a neonate with persistent cholestasis. Percutaneous liver biopsy can be performed with local anaesthetic and sedation, provided coagulation is normal.

In idiopathic neonatal hepatitis, periportal inflammatory cells are seen in conjunction with giant cells and swollen hepatocytes. Bile plugs, duct proliferation and centrazonal cholestasis are characteristic of biliary atresia. In α1-antitrypsin deficiency, diastase resistant PAS positive granular inclusions may be seen although these are usually not detected before 2–3 months of age. Liver biopsy specimens can be directly cultured for bacterial and viral infection. If the biopsy is snap frozen, specific enzyme estimation can be performed.

Laparotomy

Ultimately the diagnosis of biliary atresia may not be excluded by any of the above investigations. If the diagnosis remains a possibility, a laparotomy will be necessary.

Management

Biliary atresia

In the presence of EHBA, a Kasai operation (hepatic portoenterostomy) should be performed as a matter of urgency within a 6–8 week period from birth. This leads to a successful establishment of bile flow in up to 90 per cent of cases. When performed after 60 days the success rate is reduced to 36 per cent. Even when successful bile drainage is achieved the majority of these children develop chronic liver disease, but much more slowly than in those with persisting stasis.

Persistent cholestasis

Cholestasis resolves spontaneously in the majority of children with idiopathic neonatal hepatitis and α1-antitrypsin deficiency. In some children chronic liver disease develops. No specific treatment reverses cholestasis or prevents further liver damage. Treatment of children with chronic cholestasis is therefore aimed at obtaining maximum growth and development.

Nutritional support

In severe cholestasis, absorption of fat and fat-soluble vitamins is impaired. It is essential to maintain an adequate intake of calories. Emphasis should be based on obtaining an intake of at least 100 kcal per kg per day of ideal weight per day in children under 10 kg. Calorie requirements should never be calculated on the basis of the child's actual weight which is usually significantly below the ideal weight.

If the baby is being breastfed, this should be maintained and supplemented if necessary. In the presence of cholestasis, formulae which contain medium chain triglycerides (MCT) are optimal. These formulae can be supplemented with glucose polymers and fat. The addition of 5 per cent carbohydrate and 3 per cent fat will increase the caloric intake of a regular formula to 1 kcal per ml.

Children with chronic cholestasis are at risk of developing vitamin deficiencies. Fat soluble vitamins A, D, E and K should be supplemented together with extra amounts of water-soluble vitamins.

Choleretic agents

Pruritus is a major problem in children with chronic cholestasis. Treatment of pruritus is aimed at enchancing excretion of bile acids and is often refractory to treatment. Agents reported to be of help in children include:

1. cholestyramine, a resin which binds bile salts in the intestine, thus eliminating them in the feces. It may interfere with the absorption of fat-soluble vitamins and therefore they should be given at different times;
2. phenobarbitone, which may increase bile flow;
3. ursodeoxycholic acid, which may be effective by reducing toxic bile salts;
4. rifampicin, which may relieve pruritus by either inducing enzymes or by inhibiting bile acid uptake.

Key points

- Where jaundice persists beyond 10 days, always ask about stool and urine colour.
- α1-antitrypsin levels may be normal during stress in children with A1AT deficiency – test phenotype if the diagnosis is suspected.
- Early diagnosis and treatment greatly improves the prognosis in biliary atresia.

Useful literature

- *Liver disorders in children*, A. Mowat (Butterworth, 1994)
- Investigation of prolonged neonatal jaundice, J. Hull and D. Kelly (*Current paediatrics*, vol. 1, pp. 228–30, 1991)

33 Pallor

When parents note that their child appears pale, their main concern is that this indicates ill health or anaemia. Though acute onset pallor coupled with other signs of illness may well indicate an acute problem, the relationship between skin colour and haemoglobin level is notoriously inaccurate. Most children presenting with pallor will have a normal pale complexion and a normal haemoglobin level!

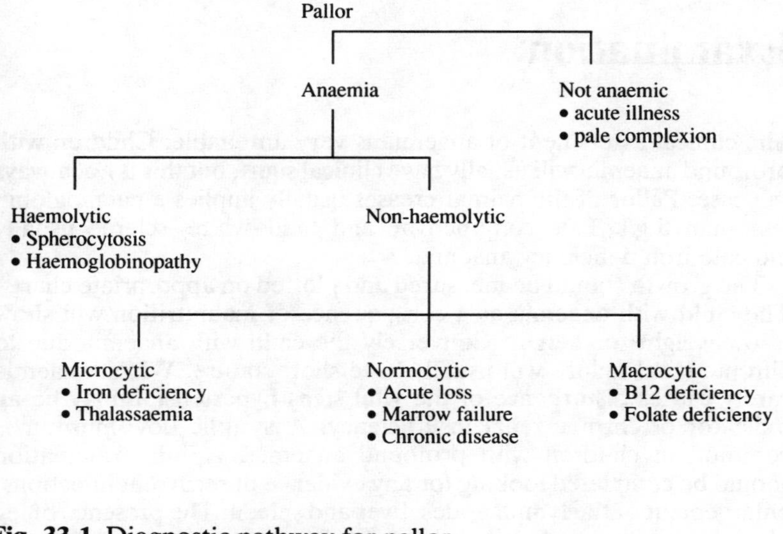

Fig. 33.1 Diagnostic pathway for pallor

History

Try to determine whether pallor is of recent onset or chronic. Pallor with onset in the last 24 hours is usually associated with acute infection, fluid loss or systemic illness. In these instances there are usually several other presenting symptoms and obvious clinical signs. Enquire as to any symptoms of anaemia such as tiredness or breathlessness. Some children with iron deficiency will eat dirt – pica. Where haemolysis is causing anaemia there may be notable episodes of jaundice or symptoms due to leg ulcers or gallstones. Acute leukaemia may present with a 2–3 week history of pallor. There may also be bone pain due to marrow infiltration, enlargement of the liver, spleen and lymph nodes or other symptoms of pancytopenia, e.g. bleeding or bacterial infection. In the past history pay particular attention to the presence of any serious neonatal jaundice or jaundice with intercurrent illnesses.

Poverty is a common antecedent of anaemia, which is usually dietary in origin. Iron deficiency anaemia is commonest in toddlers with an unbalanced diet dependent largely on cow's milk. Recurrent illnesses may also cause low grade anaemia. Family history of spherocytosis or haemoglobinopathy may be relevant. On systems review check for excessive blood loss, e.g. recurrent epistaxis, menorrhagia.

Examination

The clinical assessment of anaemia is very unreliable. Children with profound anaemia will usually have clinical signs, but this is not always the case. Pallor of the palmar creases usually implies a haemoglobin less than 5 g/l. Pale conjunctivae and 'milk-white' sclerae usually indicate iron deficiency anaemia.

The growth should be measured and plotted on appropriate charts. The child with anaemia as a consequence of malnutrition will show a low weight for height. Conversely the child with anaemia due to chronic renal failure will usually have short stature. Whilst anaemia rarely causes disturbance of the vital signs hypertension may be an indicator of chronic renal insufficiency. A systolic flow murmur is common in children with profound anaemia. A full examination should be completed looking for any evidence of recurrent infections, enlargement of the lymph nodes, liver and spleen. The presence of leg ulcers is suggestive of chronic haemolysis.

Investigation

Given that clinical assessment is so inaccurate most children will need to have a full blood count carried out. Anaemias can be divided into haemolytic and non-haemolytic anaemia. Where haemolysis is the problem there will usually be splenomegaly and jaundice – which may be intermittent. Non-haemolytic anaemias are best divided on the basis of the appearance of the red cells.

The level of haemoglobin that constitutes 'anaemia' will vary with age. Infants' haemoglobin levels are 17–20 g/l at birth, falling to the physiological nadir at 3–6 months, rising gradually thereafter. It is reasonable to take a haemoglobin of 11 grams as the lower limit of normal in children. Where the red cells are microcytic (mean corpuscular volume (MCV) less than 70) there is usually iron deficiency or more rarely thalassaemia. Anaemia with normal red cell size would imply acute bleeding, marrow infiltration or aplasia, or chronic systemic disease (e.g. renal failure, chronic arthritis). Macrocytic anaemia is usually due to vitamin B12 or folic acid deficiency.

Dietary iron deficiency is by far the commonest cause of anaemia in children. Blood loss is rarely responsible for microcytic hypochromic anaemia. Iron supplementation for a period of 2–3 months will replenish the diminished iron stores and dietary advice is mandatory. Where marrow failure due to aplastic anaemia or neoplastic infiltration is the cause of anaemia, there is usually some depression of white cells and platelets. Bone marrow examination will be necessary and specialist advice is appropriate. Macrocytic anaemias are rare. It is important to remember that MCV is physiologically elevated in early infancy. Macrocytic anaemia is most commonly associated with malabsorption, Crohn's disease or following intestinal resection.

The commonest haemolytic anaemia in Caucasians is probably congenital spherocytosis. Haemoglobinopathies and glucose-6-phosphate-dehydrogenase deficiency are much commoner in Mediterranean and Afro-Caribbean populations. Acquired haemolytic anaemia due to autoimmunity is rare in childhood.

Key points

- Pale complexion is more common than anaemia.
- Dietary iron deficiency is the main cause of anaemia.
- A diet dependent on cow's milk is likely to cause iron deficiency.
- Anaemia due to blood loss is rare.
- Jaundice, splenomegaly, and increased urinary urobilinogen indicate haemolysis.
- Clinical estimation of anaemia is very unreliable.

Useful literature

- *Handbook of haematological investigations in children*, R. Stevens (Wright, 1989)
- *Practical paediatric haematology*, R. Hinchliffe and J. Lilleyman (eds) (John Wiley, 1987)

34 Recurrent abdominal pain

Introduction

Recurrent abdominal pain is common in children. Apley's study suggested around 10 per cent of all children over 5 will complain at least three times in three months of recurrent abdominal pain severe enough to interfere with normal activities. The problem for the clinician is that in the majority of cases the diagnosis is rather soft with labels such as the periodic syndrome, abdominal migraine, psychogenic and constipation being most frequently applied. A small minority of cases have a serious underlying disorder so the difficulty for the clinician is to achieve a balance between overinvestigation and missing a diagnosis. A careful history followed by a well-directed clinical examination is the most important route to accurate diagnosis. Moreover, it will reassure the child and parents that the complaint is being taken seriously – engendering confidence in the final diagnosis.

History

The pain frequency, duration, radiation and quality should be documented and any aggravating or relieving factors noted. The single most important fact in elucidating recurrent abdominal pain is its exact location. In the case of the soft diagnoses mentioned above a child will have difficulty in precisely locating the site of the pain. When asked to use one finger to locate the pain the finger will frequently encircle the umbilicus in a rather vague way and in general the child will prefer to use the hand to identify the location. Apley said that an organic disorder was more likely the further away the pain from the umbilicus. In general this is true, but as well as distance from the umbilicus note should also be taken of the precision with which the child can locate the site of the pain.

In the case of a peptic ulcer, very frequently the child will definitely locate the pain to the epigastrium with one finger. Hepatic pain may be localised to the right hypochondrium and flank pain suggests a renal origin. Renal colic is rare in childhood and does not tend to be confused with the usual causes of recurrent abdominal pain. Haematocolpus becomes symptomatic during puberty, but there is no menstrual bleeding and pain may be of a periodic nature. Pancreatic pain may be felt in the epigastrium but may also radiate to the back. Most frequently, however, the pain will be periumbilical and rather vaguely localised.

In the past history, attention should be paid to diet and in particular, whether there has been prolonged bottle feeding and difficulty with weaning onto a more mixed diet. A low residue diet of milk and little else is the commonest predisposing factor to constipation. Dietary factors may also be important in migraine. Food allergy is a popular diagnosis with patients. Undoubtedly different foods can cause tummy upset but medical investigations are often unhelpful and even misleading. Precise dietary histories are the most helpful way to clarify the diagnosis. Lactose intolerance is a popular diagnosis in America and may well be underdiagnosed on this side of the Atlantic. Typically, there will be increased symptoms after lactose ingestion with abdominal distension, crampy abdominal pain and perhaps even audible boborygmi. Sucrose intolerance will produce similar symptoms.

Coeliac disease needs to be kept in mind especially if symptoms seem to have dated from the time of introduction of a mixed diet and if associated with poor weight gain and growth. Chronic gastroenteritis may also present with recurrent abdominal pain and food sources and preparation may need to be accurately documented. Cryptosporidium is increasingly recognised as a cause of chronic gastroenteritis and is more common in the rural population. The symptoms from giardiasis may range from mild diarrhoea to failure to thrive from malabsorption.

Family history is especially important with peptic ulcer disease. Non-abdominal causes of recurrent abdominal pain would include epilepsy, the respiratory tract and pathology of the spine. Vulvovaginitis may present with poorly localised abdominal pain. Sometimes parents will volunteer abdominal pain as the complaint although they are aware that the source of the pain is more in the perineal area. Vulvovaginitis is a common problem in young girls who have just learned toilet training independent of their parents. The usual cause of the problem is that they clean themselves forward, causing irritation and very often urinary symptoms.

Examination

Clinical examination should follow the usual paediatric routine with attention to growth and weight gain, which if suboptimal may suggest a more serious chronic disorder. The abdomen should be carefully palpated and particular note made of localised tenderness away from the umbilicus. The inguinal hernial orifices should be checked and the genitalia examined. Exclude abdominal hernias in the linea alba by palpating the midline during a sit-up. A rectal examination may be necessary. The most frequent finding would be feces in the rectum due to constipation. Careful examination of the perineum is necessary as vulvovaginitis is common in prepubertal girls. The remainder of the clinical examination should be complete as there are non-abdominal causes of recurrent abdominal pain and special attention needs to be paid to the respiratory system and the spine.

Differential diagnosis

The chief problem is often to elucidate whether or not the recurrent abdominal pain is due to constipation, abdominal migraine or a psychogenic cause. In all of these cases the pain is periumbilical and often of a rather vague nature. Constipation is a frequent cause of recurrent abdominal pain but it is difficult to be absolutely sure that this is the cause of the pain as sometimes constipation is asymptomatic and very often the bowel movement history is unreliable. There may be an apparently regular habit but yet the bowel movements are incomplete, and the result is significant constipation.

Abdominal migraine and the periodic syndrome are probably the same condition. The pain usually has a sudden onset and is of variable intensity but usually lasts a half an hour or longer. There are frequently associated symptoms which would include nausea, vomiting, headache and pallor. About 90 per cent of children with migraine have a family history of migraine and an attempt should be made to identify food triggers such as chocolate, cheese, eggs, tomatoes and citrus fruits. Prolonged fasting may also trigger migraine and is often not identified, as children may not volunteer that they have missed out on breakfast or their school lunch.

Psychological factors have long been recognised as important in recurrent abdominal pain though, like many other symptoms, the psychological factors may tend to be more secondary than primary as the underlying aetiology is better understood. Recurrent abdominal pain may accompany bulimia or anorexia nervosa and the pain may be aggravated by air swallowing.

Investigations

In the majority of cases, very few investigations are necessary. A plain film of the abdomen will confirm or refute the presence of constipation. A full blood count and differential may suggest conditions such as coeliac disease or parasitic infection if there is a significant eosinophilia. Urine culture and analysis should be done on all children with abdominal pain.

Further specific detailed investigations will then depend on the location of the pain. Epigastric pain now usually requires endoscopy and biopsy as a first line investigation rather than a barium meal. In the event of flank pain a renal ultrasound should be the initial test. Culture of the perineum may be helpful with vulvovaginitis. Most renal stones will show in a plain film of the abdomen. Detailed renal, gastrointestinal, liver, pancreatic, respiratory and neurological investigations may be required in a minority of cases.

Management

Most causes of abdominal pain are not serious. Simple constipation will often respond to an improved diet or a mild laxative such as lactulose or liquid paraffin. In abdominal migraine it may be possible to identify triggers such as foods or fasting. Children of school age will often miss out school lunches because they are too busy playing with their peers and this type of fasting may be difficult to identify. Psychogenic factors can be of importance and may well interact with the above conditions.

Undoubtedly stress can cause abdominal pain in children in much the same way as it causes headache in adults. Parents readily understand this analogy and very often this stress nowadays is from the pressure of school work and the need to achieve high grades. Lactose intolerance is not a popular diagnosis on this side of the Atlantic but is worth considering as treatment can be effective by either a low lactose diet or alternatively using lactase tablets.

Key points

- Ten per cent of school children have recurrent abdominal pain.
- Pain, localised away from the umbilicus is more likely to be organic.
- A careful history and examination may be diagnostic and therapeutic.
- Peptic ulceration is rare in childhood.

Useful literature

- *The child with abdominal pains*, J. Apley (Blackwell 1975)
- Recurrent abdominal pain in school children, M. Levine and L. Rappaport (*Paediatric clinics of North America*, vol. 31, pp. 969–91, 1984)
- Management of recurrent abdominal pain, M.S. Murphy (*Archives of diseases in childhood*, vol. 69, pp. 409–11, 1993)
- *Abdominal pain in childhood*, B. O'Donnell (Blackwell, 1985)

35 Recurrent infections

Most children suffer recurrent infections, particularly in early childhood. A healthy toddler may have at least eight mild infections per annum and those who have an older sibling at school who brings infection home may have considerably more than this number. The infections are usually viral and mostly occur during the winter months. They are shortlived and without complications in a child with an intact immune system. These children thrive well and physical examination is normal. Although there is frequently a lot of parental anxiety, no investigations are required and the parents can be reassured.

This chapter will concentrate on children with recurrent infections of unacceptable severity and/or frequency and those in whom the infections are due to unusual organisms. These cases can be divided into those in whom multiple organ systems can be infected (Fig. 35.1) and those in whom the infections are confined to a single organ. (Fig. 35.2). In the former an immune defect should be suspected whereas in the latter a structural defect in the affected organ system is the most likely cause of the problem. If, however, after extensive investigations a local cause cannot be found an immunological work-up is indicated.

Clinical evaluation of recurrent 'single site' infections

In children with recurrent infections the most common symptom complex encountered is recurrent chest infections. Asthma is the most likely underlying cause in this situation. Exacerbations of asthma in young children are usually precipitated by upper respiratory infections and the symptoms and signs may be indistinguishable from a chest infection. A chest X-ray during the exacerbation may add to the confusion, as areas of atelectasis secondary to asthma are frequently misdiagnosed as representing pneumonia. If the child is failing to thrive and/or has chronic diarrhoea the possibility of cystic fibrosis needs to be considered. Recurrent chest infections may also

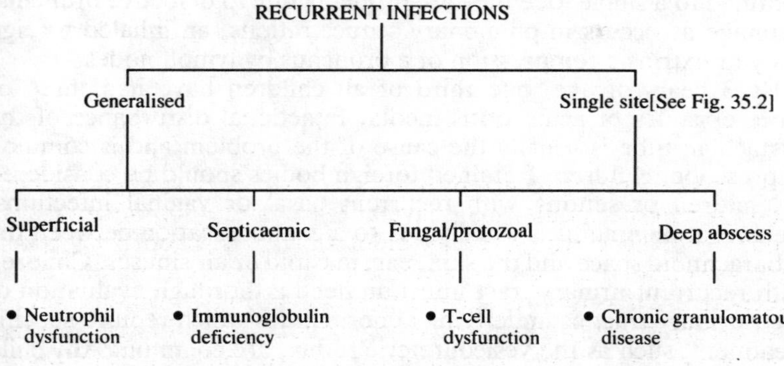

Fig. 35.1 Diagnostic possibilities for recurrent infection

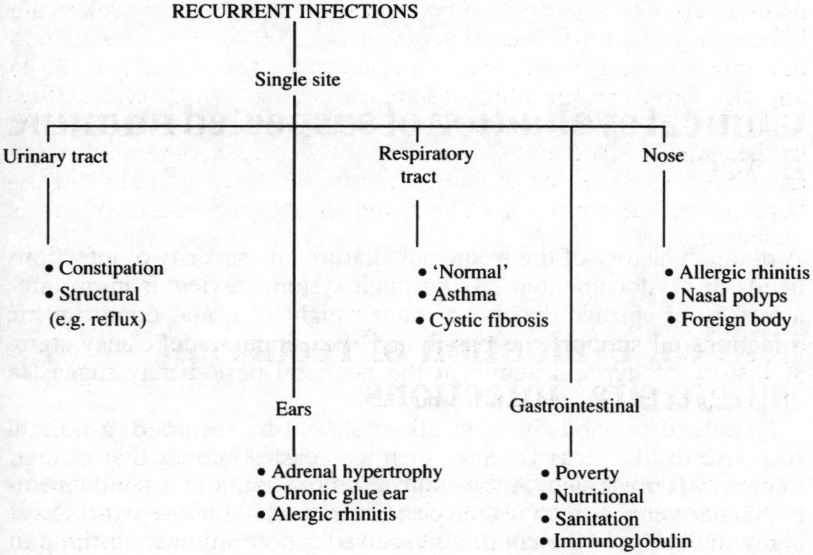

Fig. 35.2 Diagnostic possibilities for recurrent single site infection

be secondary to recurrent aspiration which in turn may be due to gastro-oesophageal reflux, H type tracheo-oesophageal fistula or a depressed cough reflex, e.g. in a child with severe cerebral palsy. Deficiency of IgA, IgG subclasses or total IgG may all give rise to recurrent sinopulmonary infection. Ciliary dyskinesia may mimic cystic fibrosis lung disease. There is usually associated sinusitis, with dextrocardia in 50 per cent of cases. If the repeated infections are confined to a single lobe they are probably due to defective bronchial drainage as occurs in pulmonary sequestrations, an inhaled foreign body or extrinsic compression of a bronchus by lymph nodes.

By 3 years of age, one third of all children have had three or more episodes of acute otitis media. Functional disturbance of the eustachian tube is usually the cause of the problem and is common in preschool children. Retained foreign bodies should be considered in children presenting with recurrent nasal or vaginal infections. Recurrent meningitis is usually due to a communication between the subarachnoid space and the skin, ear, mastoid or air sinuses. Children with recurrent urinary tract infection need a thorough evaluation of their urinary tract as underlying abnormalities which require specific treatment, such as the vesicoureteric reflux, are common. Any child with a severe skin condition, such as severe atopic eczema, is prone to repeated bacterial infection of the skin, usually due to *Staphylococcus aureus*.

Clinical evaluation of suspected immune defect

A detailed history of the frequency, nature and severity of infections needs to be documented. A thorough systems review is important: a history of chronic diarrhoea, poor weight gain and opportunistic infections all support the possibility of an immunodeficiency state. A history of hypocalcaemia in the neonatal period may suggest a diagnosis of Di George syndrome.

Details of previous immunisations should be recorded; a normal response to live virus vaccines such as measles implies that cellular immunity is preserved. A thorough enquiry about other family members is necessary as many of the primary immunodeficiency states have a genetic basis. If the child has received blood products in the past or the parents have been intravenous drug abusers the possibility of AIDS needs to be considered. A history of corticosteroid and/or cytotoxic drugs should be recorded as both may affect the immune system.

The examination should begin with an assessment of growth and nutritional status. Particular attention should be paid to lymph glands and the presence or absence of tonsils (absent in X-linked hypogammaglobulinaemia). Clubbing, skin rashes and abscesses should be noted. Telangiectasias on the conjunctivae, nasal bridge and ears are suggestive of ataxia-telangiectasia. A detailed general examination is performed with particular attention paid to the organs that have been infected in the particular case.

Investigation of suspected immune defect includes assessment of:

1. B lymphocytes which are responsible for antibody production;
2. T lymphocytes responsible for cell-mediated immunity;
3. phagocytes;
4. the complement system.

The patterns of infection associated with a defect in each system and the appropriate screening investigations are outlined in Table 35.1. B and T cell abnormalities account for the vast majority of the immune defects, whereas phagocyte and complement disorders are very rare. An effective immune response depends on a complex integration of the four systems and therefore the clinical and laboratory features of specific deficiency states may overlap. More detailed quantitative and qualitative tests are available to determine the specific immune defect in each individual case. Examples of primary immunodeficiency states affecting each system with guidelines on management are included in Table 35.2.

Paediatric acquired immunodeficiency syndrome (AIDS)

This important condition needs to be distinguished from primary immunodeficiency states. It is due to infection by the human immunodeficiency virus (HIV) and causes a combination of T and B cell defects. The majority of cases are due to vertical transmission of the virus from an infected mother, but children who received blood or blood products prior to 1985 may also have been infected. The diagnosis is made by detecting the antibody to the virus but this can be problematic in the infant as the antibody may be maternal in origin and may have been acquired by the placenta. In immunological terms the hallmark of the disease is depletion of T helper cells with reversal

Table 35.1 Investigation of immune deficiency

Immune system	**Features of deficiency**	**Screening tests**	
		Qualitative	**Quantitative**
B cells	Recurrent bacterial infections particularly due to pathogens with polysaccharide capsules, e.g. *H. influenzae, S. pneumoniae*	Immunoglobulins IgG subclases	Rubella, tetanus and polio titres post immunisations
T cells	Mucocutaneous Candidiasis *Pneumocystis carinii* pneumonia Chronic diarrhoea, failure to thrive Disseminated fungal infection	Total lymphocyte count Chest X-ray Absent thymic shadow	Delayed hypersensitivity Skin tests, e.g. Candida Phytohaemagglutinin Stimulation
Phagocytes	Skin infections Severe pyogenic infection	Differential white cell count	Nitroblue tetrazolium test (chronic granulomatous disease) Blood film for Howell–Jolly bodies (asplenia)
Complement	Recurrent meningococcal injections	Total haemolytic complement	Complement component levels

Table 35.2 Management of immune deficiency

Defective immune system	Primary immunodeficiency	Management
B cells	IgA deficiency	Symptomatic Beware of transfusion reactions with any blood products
	X linked hypogammaglobulinaemia (Bruton's)	Regular IV immunoglobulin
T cells	Di George syndrome	Thymic grafts associated with cardiac lesions
Combined T & B cells	Severe combined immuno-deficiencies	Bone marrow transplantation
Phagocytes	Asplenia	Pneumococcal, haemophilus vaccine Prophylactic penicillin for life
	Chronic granulomatous disease	Prophylactic co-trimoxazole Prompt treatment of infection ? gamma-interferon
Complement	C3 deficiency	Prompt treatment of infections

of the normal T helper:T suppressor ratio.

Almost all children with vertically acquired HIV infection develop some manifestation of infection by 12 months of age. Pneumocystic pneumonia, recurrent severe bacterial infections and failure to thrive are common. Lymphocytic interstitial pneumonitis (LIP) is a slowly progressive chronic lung disease which affects up to 50 per cent of vertically infected children. HIV encephalopathy usually presents with developmental regression and/or progressive motor signs and affects about a quarter of patients. Other manifestations of HIV infection include oral candidiasis, chronic diarrhoea, persistent parotitis, generalised lymphadenopathy and thrombocytopenia. Management consists of co-trimoxazole prophylaxis for *Pneumocystis carinii* pneumonia, appropriate treatment for specific infections as they arise and nutritional support if necessary. Specific antiretroviral therapy and regular immunoglobulin infusions have no proven role to date in the management of these children.

Key points

- Recurrent upper respiratory infections are part of normal childhood.
- Episodic asthma may be misinterpreted as recurrent chest infections.
- Infections with unusual severity, frequency, or organisms suggest immunodeficiency
- The diagnostic possibilities are very different for single site (e.g.UTI) and generalised recurrent infections.

Useful literature

- Recurrent infections, B. Herold and S. Shulman. In: *Difficult diagnosis in pediatrics*, J. Stockman (ed.) (W.B. Saunders, 1990)
- HIV infections in children, D. Gibb and M. Newell (*Archives of diseases in childhood*, vol. 67, pp. 138–41, 1992)

36 Short stature

Background

Growth is a sensitive indicator of health in childhood as normal growth occurs only if a child is healthy, adequately nourished and emotionally secure. Growth measurement is therefore an essential part of the examination or investigation of any child.

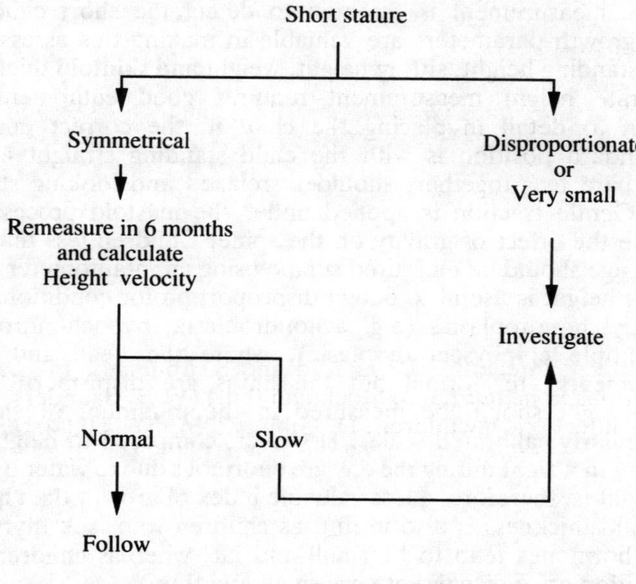

Fig. 36.1 Pathway for assessment of short stature

The definition of short stature is arbitrary, but children with the following features fall into this category:

- a height below the 3rd centile for the community;
- a height less than their genetic potential;
- a child who is falling from their centile line to a lower one.

Although most cases of short stature are due to genetic reasons or to constitutional growth delay, short stature may be the first indication of a treatable systemic illness and, as the treatment is only effective if started well before the epiphyses close at puberty, early diagnosis is essential.

The infancy-childhood-puberty (ICP) growth model analyses mathematically postnatal growth which appears to be controlled by distinct biological mechanisms. The infancy component is largely nutrition dependent, the childhood component is mostly dependent on growth hormone and the pubertal component depends on synergism between sex hormones and growth hormone.

Measuring the child

Accurate measurement is essential to detect the short child and several growth parameters are valuable in making this assessment, such as standing height, sitting height, weight and skinfold thickness.

Accurate height measurement requires good equipment and attention to detail in placing the child in the correct position. The standard position is with the child standing straight against a wall, bare feet together, shoulders relaxed and looking straight ahead. Gentle traction is applied under the mastoid processes to eliminate the effect of gravity on the spine. Children less than two years of age should be measured supine using an infantometer.

Sitting height is useful to detect disproportion for conditions such as the dyschondroplasias (e.g. achondroplasia, hypochondroplasia and multiple epiphyseal dysplasia), where the head and trunk measurements are normal but the limbs are disproportionately short. Weight should be measured in the minimum of clothing on a regularly calibrated scales. However, compared to height, the variations in weight during the day are enormous due to water balance and weight is, therefore, a less valuable index of growth than height.

Skinfold thickness is also useful, as children who lack thyroid or growth hormones tend to be small and fat, whereas children with malnutrition or coeliac disease are small and thin.

Good measuring equipment is essential for measuring height

velocity as the normal growth rate is only 4–6 cm per year between the ages of approximately 3 and 10 years. The most accurate equipment is a wall mounted Harpenden stadiometer, however, less expensive portable equipment is also available. The measurement is evaluated by plotting the reading on the appropriate centile chart for the community.

The parents' height is also important in the assessment of a child, as height is genetically inherited. It is best to measure both parents, as wives tend to overestimate their husband's height. The height of both parents is plotted on the chart at 19 years with the following adjustment made for the sex of the child: 12.5 cm is subtracted from the father's height if the child is a girl; and 12.5 cm is added to the mother's height if the child is a boy. The mid-point between these two measurements is called the midparental height and the child's centile line should fall within 8.5 cm either side of this centile line. Any child whose centile line is more than 8.5 cm below the midparental line may not be achieving their full genetic potential.

Growth velocity

The most valuable measurement of growth is the height velocity which is the gain in height over a period of time. In order to determine the height velocity two measurements are needed, ideally at a year's interval, as there are seasonal variations in growth; children tend to grow more in the spring than they do in the autumn and winter and intercurrent mild illness may cause a transient fall in height velocity followed by a catch-up period after recovery from the illness. Poor height velocity is an indicator of an organic cause which should be sought, whereas the child with a normal height velocity is a normal child with normal variant short stature. Growth standards are now available for a variety of growth disorders, e.g. Turner syndrome, Down's syndrome and achondroplasia.

Bone age

An X-ray of the hand and wrist illustrates the maturity and bone growth or bone age which is an indicator of growth potential. The child with genetic short stature will have a bone age consistent with his chronological age, whereas a child with constitutional growth delay or a systemic disorder will have a delayed bone age indicating potential for catch-up. In children under the age of 18 months knees and ankles are used.

Causes of short stature

Normal variant

In the normal variant group constitutional growth delay is the most common cause. These are the slow developing children who are small and have a late puberty. They therefore go on growing for a longer period before their pubertal growth spurt, so that they catch up and have a good normal adult height. There is often a family history of growth delay or late puberty. The two other main causes are familial or genetic short stature where either parent is short and intrauterine growth retardation, where the child is born small for gestational age, then grows with a normal height velocity and has a short adult height usually within the normal range.

Pathological Causes

Approximately 25 per cent of children referred by a paediatric endocrine clinic with short stature have a pathological cause. They usually have clinical signs or a poor height velocity which may be the major diagnostic clue. They require early investigation so that the cause can be determined and early treatment instituted where possible. The main pathological causes of short stature are:

- nutritional deficiency – worldwide, protein-calorie malnutrition is the most common cause of growth failure;
- chronic infection involving any organ system may result in poor growth;
- malabsorption, e.g. coeliac or other gastrointestinal disorders such as Crohn's disease or ulcerative colitis;
- chromosomal disorders such as Turner syndrome where short stature may be the only clinical feature and other syndromes such as Noonan's syndrome which occurs in both boys and girls;
- skeletal dysplasias usually have disproportionate body measurements and may have other clinical features also;
- chronic illness such as renal disorders or congenital heart disease may inhibit growth;
- psychosocial deprivation may present solely as short stature associated with poor height velocity;

- endocrine causes – include growth hormone deficiency, hypothyroidism and glucocorticoid excess. These children grow with a poor height velocity and have a greater weight and skinfold thickness percentile than that for height.

History

A full medical and social history should be taken. This must include birthweight, developmental milestones, growth rate and specific questions related to aetiology of short stature listed in Table 36.1.

A family history should include height of parents and siblings and also timing of puberty together with a history of any general illnesses.

Physical examination

A complete physical examination is required including growth measurements to assess height, weight, sitting height, skinfold

Table 36.1 Causes of short stature

Normal variant
Familial or genetic short stature
Intrauterine growth retardation
Constitutional growth delay
Pathological causes
Nutritional deficiency
Chronic infection
Malabsorption
Chromosomal disorders
Skeletal dysplasias
Chronic illness
Psychosocial deprivation
Endocrine:
• growth hormone deficiency
• hypothyroidism
• glucocorticoid excess

thickness and staging of puberty, if signs are present. Blood pressure, fundi and visual fields must be assessed and other more specific findings sought, such as the presence of small external genitalia in a male (suggesting pituitary deficiency), café au lait spots or freckling (suggesting neurofibromatosis), dysmorphic features, signs of malabsorption, renal disease or congenital heart disease.

Investigations

Investigations of poor growth are summarised in Table 36.2.

Growth hormone tests

The diagnosis of growth hormone deficiency requires the presence of short stature, poor height velocity, ideally over a 12-month period, and low serum growth hormone levels. Growth hormone is secreted in a pulsatile manner approximately 4-hourly, most frequently during sleep, and in between times there are very low blood levels. A random growth hormone level is therefore of little value and a provocation test is required.

The stimulus used can be physiological or pharmacological.

Table 36.2 Investigation of poor growth

Bone age
Karyotype (girls)

Specific investigations (when indicated):

- Full blood count, ESR
- Electrolytes, creatinine, bicarbonate calcium, phosphate, alkaline phosphatase and liver enzymes.
- Gastrointestinal, to include stool culture, jejunal biopsy if coeliac disease suspected and barium studies and endoscopy may be indicated to diagnose Crohn's disease or ulcerative colitis.
- Endocrine tests:
  - TSH and thyroxine levels
  - diurnal cortisol levels
  - growth hormone provocation tests
- Radiology: skull X-ray and computerised tomography to exclude a brain tumour in growth hormone deficiency.

Exercise is a physiological stimulus and blood is taken 20 minutes after controlled exercise. If the serum growth hormone level rises to 15 mU/l or greater the growth hormone level is considered normal and if the blood level is less than 15 mU/l the child proceeds to a pharmacological test.

Pharmacological stimulation tests are not without danger and must be performed with very close medical supervision, and laboratory results must be interpreted with caution due to interassay and interlaboratory variability problems.

Pharmacological stimulation tests include:

1. Insulin hypoglycaemia test which must have a doctor in attendance, good intravenous access, hydrocortisone and 10 per cent glucose immediately available. Insulin 0.1 mg/kg bodyweight is given intravenously and blood is taken at 15 minute intervals for 90 minutes; the blood sugar should fall to 2.2 mmol/l or lower; this test should only be performed in specialised growth assessment centres because of the risks of profound hypoglycaemia or rebound hyperglycaemia.
2. L-dopa propranolol;
3. Glucagon;
4. Clonidine.

Other physiological tests include a 24 hour growth hormone profile taking blood at 20 minute intervals; however, this is traumatic for the child and involves considerable clinical, laboratory and staff time. Urine growth hormone levels can be estimated, but reports vary as to their accuracy. Insulin-like growth factor binding protein 3 (IGF BP3) is closely related to GH secretion and may prove to be a useful test in the future.

In patients who are in the immediate prepuberty age range with bone ages in excess of 10 years, or girls with little or no signs of puberty, there is often a blunting of the growth hormone response to conventional provocation. The use of a single intramuscular dose of 100 mg of mixed testosterone esters in boys 3–5 days before the growth hormone provocation, and in girls the administration of ethinyloestradiol in a daily dose of 100 μg/day for three days prior to the test, will usually produce a normal response in those who are not growth hormone deficient.

Treatment

Treatment aims to correct the underlying problem where possible (e.g.

gluten free diet for coeliac disease, thyroxine in hypothyroidism). The earlier the treatment the better the final height.

Growth hormone is given as a daily (bedtime) subcutaneous infection in a dose of 0.5–1.0 unit/kg/week, in case of GH deficiency

Many girls with Turner syndrome improve height velocity and final height with growth hormone treatment. However, the optimal dosage and age for starting treatment have not yet been established. Apart from Turner syndrome there is no evidence that growth hormone treatment will improve final height in children who are not growth hormone deficient.

The potential side-effects of growth hormone treatment are glucose intolerance, hyperinsulinism, hyperlipidaemia or hypertension. Leukaemia may be more common in growth hormone deficient children treated with growth hormone, but there is currently no evidence causally linking treatment with leukaemia or evidence that tumour recurrence or second tumours are more common.

Constitutional growth delay

Boys who are very distressed by their late puberty may be given oxandrolone 0.05 mg/kg/day for 6–12 months until the endogenous growth spurt commences.

Psychological

The treatment of short stature should aim not only to promote growth and final height but also to alleviate any psychosocial problems. The child and family require early psychological counselling and the child requires encouragement and a supportive environment. Short children must be treated in accordance with their age and not their size; tall children have been shown to mature earlier as they are given more responsibility, whereas small children mature later as they are treated as being less able.

Conclusion

Growth is a sensitive indicator of good health in childhood and height measurement is, therefore, a vital part of any clinical examination. Where there is a treatable cause of short stature, the earlier the diagnosis and treatment the better the final adult height. If the cause is untreatable, it is important to discuss the problem with the parents and the child in order to minimise or avoid psychological disturbances that may result.

Ideally, every child should have an accurate height measurement at not later than the age of 5 years. This should be done by the family doctor or the school medical officer. If this is below the 3rd centile for the average developer, referral to a growth clinic should be considered. The child will then have a full history and physical examination and if this is abnormal he will be investigated immediately. However, if the history and examination are normal he will be measured again after 1 year with a stadiometer. If at this time his velocity is poor, he will be fully investigated. Alternatively if the velocity is normal there is no need for further follow-up.

Key points

- Stature can be measured at one visit, growth requires serial measurements.
- The commonest cause of a short child is short parents.
- Short, fat children may have an endocrine problem.
- Accurate serial height measurements are the most important indicator of growth hormone status.
- Delay in diagnosis of growth hormone insufficiency reduces attainable adult height – growth hormone treatment can give normal growth but cannot catch up on 'lost' growth.

Useful literature

- The management of short stature, C. Brook, P. Hindmarsh and P. Smith. In: *Clinical paediatric endocrinology*, 2nd edition, C. Brook (ed.) (Blackwell, 1989)
- Normal growth and its endocrinology, P. Hindmarsh and C. Brook. In: *Clinical paediatric endocrinology*, 2nd edition, C. Brook (ed.) (Blackwell, 1989)
- The design and use of growth standards, H. Hoey (*Growth matters*, vol. 7, pp. 2–4, 1991)
- Psychosocial aspects of short stature, H. Hoey (*Journal of pediatric endocrinology*, 1993, p. 6)

- Endocrine gland disorders, C. Kelnar. In: *Forfar and Arneil's textbook of paediatrics*, 4th edition, A. Campbell and N. McIntosh (eds) (Churchill Livingstone, 1992)

37 Skin rash

Introduction

Skin rashes are extremely common in children and one of the main reasons for consultations in primary care. The types and the causes of rashes are numerous. This section will concentrate on the commonest and most important presentations.

Rashes can generally be divided into acute and chronic. Rashes with onset in the preceding day are frequently associated with infectious diseases or immediate allergic reactions. Rashes which have been present for some time can be either generalised or localised. The differential diagnosis of a chronic rash in infancy is quite different from that in older children and these will be considered separately.

It is important to be clear on the terminology so that one can accurately describe a rash and compare it with definitions in textbooks. A macule is a red spot, a papule is an elevated spot, a vesicle is an elevated spot containing fluid. A petechial rash does not blanch on pressure. Scratching would tend to suggest a pruritic rash. Colour atlases of dermatology are invaluable in sorting out rarer conditions. Pattern recognition becomes easier with clinical experience.

Acute rash

History

The approach to the child with onset of rash in the preceding 24 hours follows along the lines of general clinical assessment. Try to define the precise onset and evolution of the rash and any associated symptoms at onset. Define whether there was a febrile prodrome or contact with infectious disease. A detailed medication history is important and also details as to previous episodes of skin rash.

Clinical examination

The first priority is to detect the child with serious infection who presents with skin rash. Children with meningococcal septicaemia typically develop a petechial rash, though this may be macular for a period of time. The presence of fever and signs of general toxicity should alert one to this possibility.

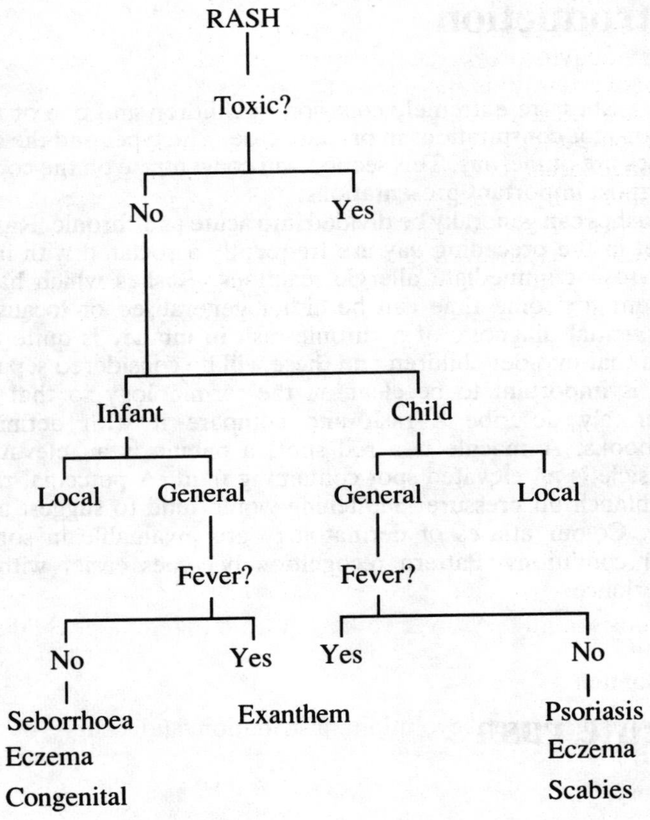

Fig. 37.1 Diagnostic pathway for skin rash

A full description of the rash and its distribution should be carefully documented. The nature and particular focus of the general examination will depend on the nature of the rash described. For instance, the child with a maculopapular rash and fever may well have measles so that Koplik spots, evidence of conjunctivitis, pharyngitis and respiratory infection would be sought. Where the rash has been provoked by ampicillin, the possibility of infectious mononucleosis is raised and particular attention should be paid to detecting lymphadenopathy and splenomegaly.

Diagnosis in infants

The diagnosis of acute rashes is largely clinical. Laboratory investigations are of little value. The major 'exanthems' are varicella, measles, rubella, roseola, parvovirus, scarlet fever and staphylococcal scalded skin. In addition, where ampicillin is inadvertently administered to patients with infectious mononucleosis a 'measles-like' rash develops in approximately 90 per cent.

A purpuric rash should immediately raise the possibility of meningococcal septicaemia. As detailed in the section on bleeding and bruising, purpura may also be due to thrombocytopenia, vasculitic processes or raised venous pressure due to prolonged coughing, choking or application of a tourniquet.

Urticarial rashes can develop acutely and are generally allergic or photosensitive. In many cases it is not possible to be precise regarding the allergic trigger.

Chronic rash

Children with rash for more than 24 hours are more likely to present in primary care or in a hospital outpatient setting. The differential diagnosis in infancy is very different from that in later childhood.

Evaluation

Record the onset, evolution, distribution and course of the skin rash. Enquire as to whether there were any precipitating events and whether there is pruritis. A previous history of rash is clearly important. Enquire as to the presence of other affected individuals in the house or in recent contact. Record previous usage of creams and applications as these may modify the appearance of the rash.

Diagnosis

Chronic rashes in infancy can divided into normal, inflammatory, infectious and congenital.

Normal Milia – small white spots around the nose, due to prominent sebaceous glands, are normal in the newborn. Neonatal urticaria occurs in over a third of infants typically with onset in the first week and clearing spontaneously thereafter. The aetiology is unclear and spontaneous recovery always occurs. Neonatal acne is very similar in appearance to teenage acne and often follows at 2–3 weeks of age. The appearance may persist for several weeks but again spontaneous complete recovery is the rule.

Inflammatory Inflammatory conditions would include seborrhoeic dermatitis and eczema. Seborrhoeic dermatitis is now known to be due to infection with a lipophilic yeast - *Pityrosporum ovale*, often associated with poor hygiene. The infant will develop the triad of 'cradle cap', napkin rash which looks uniform and salmon pink, and a flaking rash around the eyebrows and behind the ears. The axillae may also be affected. The child is usually not disturbed by the rash and treatment with a combination of antifungal and mild hydrocortisone treatment with local hygiene usually effects a complete recovery.

Infantile eczema usually begins at around three months of age and typically starts at the sides of the face before extending down to the trunk. In contrast to seborrhoeic dermatitis the rash is itchy and the child is frequently distressed and miserable. In chronic cases there is often secondary infection due to scratching and lichenification in areas severely affected. In infancy occasional patients benefit from an exclusion diet. In general, management is with a combination of parent education, emollients, topical corticosteroids, antihistamines and antibiotics. The safety of mild topical steroids should be made clear to parents

Napkin rash is common and is usually due to 'ammoniacal dermatitis'. In this case the rash is usually worst in the distribution of urine passage and on the 'convexities' of the skin folds. Attention to hygiene, frequent nappy changes and application of a barrier cream are usually curative. The napkin rash of seborrheoic dermatitis is usually uniform in distribution and follows a 'bathing trunk' pattern. Candida may cause napkin rash in isolation or commonly causes superinfection of other nappy rash. Where candida is dominant, lesions are more evident in the 'concavities' of the skin folds and there is often a peeling edge to the rash with satellite lesions. Topical treatment with antifungal agents is appropriate.

Infectious The major infection causing chronic skin rash in infancy and in older children is scabies. The primary infection may be in the hands or feet and the generalised papulo-vesicular, pruritic rash is felt to be due to hypersensitivity. This rash may be particularly difficult to recognise. Clues in the history will include chronicity, resistence to topical corticosteroids and history of affected siblings or parents. Attention to home hygiene and application of benzyl benzovate or crotamiton are usually effective. All family members should be treated.

Congenital Congenital dermatoses are rare but can be potentially lethal. Bullous lesions in the newborn period may be due to staphylococcal sepsis but where the child is well, recurrent lesions on pressure points would suggest the possibility of epidermolysis bullosa. Several other skin rashes may be associated with neurological problems – the so-called 'neuro-cutaneous' syndromes.

Older children

Chronic rashes in older children may be generalised or local. Generalised conditions would include eczcema, which has persisted, and psoriasis. Local skin rashes are far more common and are often infectious.

Local rashes

Warts are caused by a papilloma virus. These are very common in children and will disappear spontaneously. Where warts are troublesome they may be treated with topical applications or cryotherapy. Molluscum contagiosum is a wartlike lesion caused by a pox virus. The lesions may be single or multiple, are raised and have central umbilication. Spontaneous recovery is the rule.

Rashes around the mouth may be due to staphylococcal or herpes simplex infection. Clinical differentiation is straightforward, herpetic lesions are vesicular and often affect the mucus membranes. Tinea corporis will cause patchy, typically circular lesions with a spreading edge on any part of the body. Examination of scrapings under microscopy is often diagnostic and treatment with topical or, in resistant cases, oral antifungal agents is curative. Infection with animal fungus may cause a very vigorous inflammatory reaction. The 'kerion' resulting from cattle ringworm may be mistaken for a subcutaneous abscess on the scalp. Treatment needs to be carried on beyond apparent cure to prevent relapse.

Troublesome rash on the feet is usually due to tinea pedis. In this case lesions are most prominent in the interdigital spaces and treatment with antifungal agents is appropriate. Juvenile plantar dermatosis is a frictional dermatitis seen with increased frequency in young children who wear 'trainers'. The affected area becomes red, dry, cracked and painful and may bleed. Management involves a change in footwear and treatment with moisturisers and mild steroids.

Acne is extremely common in teenagers and can viewed as a normal developmental skin process in the majority. Where lesions are extensive and causing morbidity treatment is indicated. Local applications have a limited role. Prolonged courses of antibiotics such as erythromycin or tetracycline are effective in moderate cases. Where lesions are severe or cystic, treatment with retinoids may be contemplated but this is best done under specialist supervision.

Generalised

The common rashes in children are eczema and psoriasis. The management of eczema follows along similar lines to infancy. The management of psoriasis is evolving. Coal tar preparations, dithranol and ultraviolet treatments all have a role.

If the clinical pattern does not fall into an obvious category, consult your textbook!

Key points

- Napkin rash can be ammoniacal, candidal or seborrhoeic.
- A papulo-vesicular pruritic rash is usually due to scabies.
- Severe eczema in infancy responds to diet in about 10 per cent of cases.
- Topical 1 per cent hydrocortisone is safe.
- Treatment of fungal skin infection needs to be prolonged beyond apparent cure.

Useful literature

- *Essential paediatric dermatology*, J. Verbov (Clinical Press, 1988)
- *Colour textbook of paediatric dermatology*, W. Weston and A. Lane (Mosby Year Book, 1991)

Index

ABC of resuscitation
  collapsed child, 32–3
  poisoning, 98
  seizures, 105
Abdomen
  pain in, 233–7
  physical examination
    crying child, 54–5
    hepatobiliary disease, 80, 221
    vomiting child, 20
  ultrasound in liver disease, 84
Abscess, brain, 202
Absences, 193
Abuse (child), 37–45
  emotional, 40–1
  management, 43–4
  physical, *see* Non-accidental injury
  sexual, 42–3, 44, 160
Acetaminophen, *see* Paracetamol
Acetylcysteine in paracetamol poisoning, 102
Acid, caustic, poisoning by, 100
Acne
  neonatal, 258
  teenage, 260
Acute illness observation scales (AIOS) in febrile child, 66, 67, 68
Adolescents/teenagers
  acne, 260
  intentional poisoning, 97
  puberty, *see* Puberty
Adrenal hyperplasia, congenital, precocious puberty in, 129
β-Adrenoceptor agonists in asthma, 139
Adsorbents in diarrhoeal illness, 16
AIDS, 241–4
Airway
  assessment
    collapsed child, 32
    poisoned child, 98
    seizures, 105
  obstruction, stridor due to, 119–23
Albumin levels in liver disease, 82, 223
Albuminuria, 94
Alimentary tract, *see* Gastrointestinal tract *and specific regions*
Alkali, caustic, poisoning by, 100
Alkaline phosphatase levels in hepatobiliary disease, 82, 223
Alpha-1-antitrypsin deficiency, 84, 86, 223
Aminotransferase levels, 81–2, 221–3
Ammoniacal dermatitis, 258
Anaemia, 229–32
  assessment, 230
  investigation, 231
Androgens, adrenal, precocious puberty caused by excessive, 129
Anoxic events, reflex, 194
Antibacterial drugs
  cystic fibrosis, 166–7
  diarrhoeal illness, 16
  pneumonia, 63
Antibodies, auto-, in autoimmune chronic active hepatitis, 84
Anticonvulsants, 109, 197
Antidiarrhoeal drugs, 16
Antiprotozoal drugs, diarrhoeal illness, 16
Antipyretics, 69

Antisocial behaviour, 146–7
α1-Antitrypsin deficiency, 84, 86, 223
Antitussives, 50
Anus
  in constipation, inspection, 159–60
  reflex dilatation, 160
Aortic valve lesions, 207, 208, 209, 211, 212, 213
Apnoea, 195
Arrhythmia, cardiac, *see* Tachycardia
Arteries
  access in collapsed child, 33
  blood gas sampling in dyspnoea, 61–2
Arthritis, septic, 89
Aspirin, contraindication, 69
Asplenia, 243
Asthma, 135–41
  acute, 48, 59–60
  exacerbation by infection, 238–40
  outpatient management, 135–41
  symptoms, 48, 59–60
Atresia, biliary, 225
Atrial septal defect, 213
Attention deficit disorders, 147
Auscultation, cardiac, 206–13
Autoimmune chronic active hepatitis, 83–4, 85

B cell deficiency, 241, 242, 243
Bacterial infection (in general), diarrhoea due to, 10
Bacterial pneumonia, 47
Bacterial sepsis, 67
Bacterial tracheitis, 121
Bacteriology, *see* Microbiology
Battered baby syndrome, 37, *see also* Non-accidental injury
Bedwetting, *see* Enuresis
Behavioural problem(s)/ syndrome(s), 142–8
  colic as, 56
Beta-agonists in asthma, 139
Biliary disease, neonatal, 217–28
  management, 226–7
Bilirubin, accumulation, *see* Hyperbilirubinaemia
Biochemistry
  diarrhoeal illness, 153
  seizure patient, 107–8
Biopsy
  liver, 85, 225–6
  renal, 75
Bleeding/haemorrhage, 25–31
  generalised, 26
  single-site, 26
Bleeding time, 28
Blood
  gases, sampling in dyspnoea, 61–2
  tests (in general), *see* Haematology
  in urine, *see* Haematuria
Blood supply, *see* Arteries; Circulation; Veins
Bone
  age, measurement, 247–8
  fractures, *see* Fractures
  infection, limping due to, 87, 89
  scans, limping child, 89
Bowel, *see* Intestine
Brain abscess, 202, *see also entries under* Cerebral; Head; Intracranial
Breast development, premature, 131
Breathholding attacks, 146, 195
Breathing
  assessment/management
    collapsed child, 32–3
    poisoned child, 98
  difficulties, 58–64, 119–23
Bronchiectasis, 48, 50
Bronchiolitis, acute
  management, 63–4
  symptoms, 60
Bronchitis, laryngotracheo-, 121, 122
Bronchodilators in asthma, 136–7, 138, 139
Bruising, 25–31
  in liver disease, 79
  non-accidental, 25, 26, 38–9
Bruton's disease, 243
Burns, non-accidental, 39

C3 deficiency, 243
Calcium blood levels, seizures with low, 107

Calculi, renal, 75
Candida infections of skin, 258
Cardiomyopathy, obstructive, 212
hypertrophic, 212
Cardiovascular system in cholestatic neonates, 221, *see also entries under* Heart
Care Order, 44
Catheterisation, cardiac, 214–15
Caustic acid/alkalis, poisoning by, 100
Cerebral disorders (in general), *see also* Brain *and entries under* Neurological
collapse due to, 35
vomiting due to, 21, 23
Cerebral palsy, 173–4
Ceruloplasmin levels, 83
Charcoal, activated, in poisoning, 99, 100
Chest infections, *see* Infections
Child Protection Agency, 43, 44
Chlamydial pneumonia, 63
Cholangiopancreatography, endoscopic retrograde, 85
Choleretic agents, 227
Cholestasis, 217–28
intrahepatic and extrahepatic, differentiation, 221–5
neonatal, 217–28
persistent, 226
Cholestyramine, 227
Chorionic gonadotrophin, human, test employing, 132
Chromosomal disorders causing short stature, 248
Chronic disease, short stature in, 248
Circulation
assessment/management
collapsed child, 33
poisoned child, 99
seizures, 105
failure in diarrhoeal illness, 12
Clotting, *see* Coagulation
Coagulation/clotting
disorders, 28, 30
tests, 29
Coagulation/clotting factors
abnormal levels, 29, 223
replacement therapy, 30
Coeliac disease, 152, 189
Colestasis, neonatal, 217–28
Colic, infantile, 56–7
cause, 56
'malignant', 57
Colitis, ulcerative, 152
Collapsed child, 32–6
Complement deficiency, 242, 243
in autoimmune chronic active hepatitis, 84
Compliance
in asthma therapy, 136
in diabetes management, 177
Computed tomography, seizure patient, 109, 196
Congenital adrenal hyperplasia, precocious puberty in, 129
Congenital dermatoses, 259
Congenital heart disease, *see also specific types of disease*
dyspnoea, 60
education, 215
failure to thrive, 191
murmurs, 208
Congenital stridor, 120
Constipation, 155–62, 235
causes, 157
Constitutional growth delay, 132, 252
Convulsions, *see* Seizures
Co-operation, gaining
of crying child, 54
of parents of crying child, 54
Copper values, 81, 83
Corticosteroids, *see* Steroids
Cough, 46–51
acute, 47–8
chronic, 48–9
Counselling of parents in sudden infant death, 114
Crohn's disease, 153
Cromoglycate in asthma, 138, 139
Croup
coughing and, 47
dyspnoea in, 58–9
Crying (persistent/prolonged episodes), 52–7
acute, 52–5
causes, 53–4

chronic, 55–7
quality, on Acute Illness Observation Scale, 68
Cutaneous problems, *see* Skin
Cyanotic attacks, 194
Cyanotic heart disease, 202
Cyproterone acetate in precocious puberty, 131
Cystic fibrosis, 48, 151, 163–8, 224
cough in, 48
diarrhoea in, 151
sweat test, 224

Death, *see* Infanticide; Sudden infant death
Defaecation, normal sequence, 155–6
Dehydration, diarrhoea-related, 11–12, 12, 13
management, 14, 15
Dermatitis/eczema, 260
ammoniacal, 258
infantile, 258
seborrhoeic, 258
Dermatoses, *see* Dermatitis; Rash; Skin
Destructive behaviour, 146–7
Development, 169–75
delayed, 169–75
milestones, 171
Di George syndrome, 243
Diabetes mellitus, 176–9
Diarrhoea, 9–17, 149–54
acute, 9–17
aetiology, 9–10, 10, 11
risk factors, 11
chronic, 149–54
Diastolic murmurs, 208
systolic and, 208
Diazepam with seizures, 109
Diet, *see* Nutrition
Digestive tract, *see* Gastrointestinal tract *and specific regions*
Diplegia, spastic, 174
Disseminated intravascular coagulation, 30
Doppler studies of cardiac blood flow, 214
Dreams, frightening, 145
Drugs, *see also specific (types of) drugs*
accidental and intentional (non-therapeutic) ingestion, *see* Poisoning
compliance in asthma, 136
in nocturnal enuresis, 184
reactions, 194–5
Ductus arteriosus, patent, 209
Dyspnoea, 58–64
Dysrhythmia, cardiac, *see* Tachycardia

Ear infections, 240
Eating problems, 143, *see also* Feeding; Nutrition
Echocardiography, 214
Eczema, *see* Dermatitis
Education, patient/parents, 5–6
with murmurs, 215
with seizures, 196–7
EEG, seizure patient, 109, 196
Effusions, pericardial, 61
Ehlers-Danlos syndrome, 28
Eisenmenger syndrome, 208
Ejection systolic murmurs, 210, 211
Electroencephalography, seizure patient, 109, 196
Emesis, *see* Vomiting
Emotional abuse, 40–1
Encopresis, 58
Endocrinology, *see* Hormones
Endoscopic retrograde cholangiopancreatography, 85
Enteropathy
gluten (coeliac disease), 152, 189
protein-losing, 94
Enuresis, nocturnal, 180–5
primary, 181, 182
secondary, 181, 182
Enzymes, hepatic, 81–2, 221–3
Epiglottitis, 59, 62, 122
investigations, 62, 122
management, 122
signs/symptoms, 59, 120, 121
Epilepsy, 193
seizures in, condition mimicking, 194–5
Exanthema, 257

Exercise, murmurs in response to, 213
Eye signs/symptoms in jaundice/hepatobiliary disease, 80, 220, 222

Faecal analysis, *see* Stools
Failure to thrive, 40–1, 186–91
Fainting (syncope), 195
Fallot's tetralogy, 208
Febrile illness, *see* Fever
Feeding patterns, failure to thrive and, 187, *see also* Eating problems
Fever, 65–71
  convulsions precipitated by, 108, 193
  headache and, 200
First aid, *see also* Resuscitation
  collapsed child, 32–3
  seizures, 105
Fistula, tracheo-oesophageal, 48, 50
Fits, *see* Seizures
Fluid, interstitial, excessive, *see* Oedema
Fluid therapy
  in diarrhoeal illness, 14, 15
  intravenous, *see* Intravenous fluid therapy
  oral, 14, 15
  in shock, 34
Food poisoning, toxin-mediated, 10
Foreign body inhalation, 62, 120, 122
Fractures
  detection, 89
  non-accidental, 38, 39
Fructose intolerance, 224
Fungal skin infection, 258, 259–60
Funny turns, 193

Galactosaemia, 224
Gamma glutamyltransferase/ transpeptidase levels in hepatobiliary disease, 82, 223
Gas, arterial blood, sampling in dyspnoea, 61–2
Gastroenteritis
  acute, 10
  chronic, 234
Gastrointestinal tract problems (in general) in cystic fibrosis, 164
Gastro-oesophageal reflux, *see* Reflux
Genital examination
  crying child, 54–5
  sexual abuse, 43
Giardiasis, 151
Glucose (sugar), blood, seizure patient, 107, *see also* Hypoglycaemia
γ-Glutamyltransferase/ transpeptidase levels in hepatobiliary disease, 82, 223
Gluten enteropathy (coeliac disease), 152, 189
Glycaemic control, 176
Gonadal dysfunction/failure, 132
Gonadotrophin
  deficiency, 132
  ectopic production, 129
  human chorionic, test employing, 132
Gonadotrophin-releasing hormone agonist/analogues in precocious puberty, 131
Grand mal seizures, 193
Granulomatous disease, chronic, 243
Growth
  constitutional delay, 132, 252
  measurement, 245, 246–7
  poor
    chronic diarrhoea and, 151–2
    in cystic fibrosis, 164
    investigation, 250
Growth hormone
  administration, 252
    side-effects, 252
  deficiency, tests, 250–1
Gut, *see* Gastrointestinal tract *and specific regions*

Haematology
  in diarrhoeal illness, 153
  in hepatobiliary disease, 81, 222
  in seizure patients, 108
Haematuria, 72–6
  causes, 74
Haemolytic anaemia, 231

Haemophilus influenzae, 63
  type B, 59, 121
Haemorrhage, *see* Bleeding
Hand signs in liver disease, 79
Head injuries, non-accidental, 38, *see also entries under* Brain; Intracranial
Headache, 199–204
  acute, 200–1
  migrainous, *see* Migraine
  recurrent, 201–3
Heart
  disease/disorders, 60–1, 205–16
    collapse due to, 35
    congenital, *see* Congenital heart disease
    cyanotic, 202
    dyspnoea in, 60–1
    in jaundiced neonates, 221
  murmurs, *see* Murmurs
  sounds, 206–7
Height
  measurement, 246, 246–7
  parents', 247
Hepatic disease/tests, *see* Liver
Hepatitis
  chronic active autoimmune, 83–4, 85
  infectious (in general), 23
  neonatal, 225
  viral, 82–3
    type A, 82, 85
    type B, 82, 85
    type C, 83, 85
    type D, 83
Hepatolenticular degeneration (Wilson's disease), 83, 85–6
Hess test, 28
Hip joint problems, 87–8, 89, 90
Hirschprung's disease, 160, 161
History-taking, principles, 2, 3
HIV infection/AIDS, paediatric, 241–4
Hormones
  in jaundiced neonates, disorders, 224–5
  puberty and
    abnormal, 129, 132
    normal, 127–8
  short stature due to disorders of, 248–9, 250
HPV (human papilloma virus), 259
Human chorionic gonadotrophin test, 132
Human papilloma virus, 259
Hydration
  abnormally low level, *see* Dehydration
  on Acute Illness Observation Scale, status, 68
  therapy, *see* Fluid therapy
Hyperactivity, 147
Hyperbilirubinaemia, conjugated and unconjugated, 77, 78
  causes, 78, 217–18, 219
  differentiation, 221–5
  neonatal, 217–28
Hypernatraemia, seizures in, 107
Hypernatraemic dehydration, 13
Hypertension, intracranial, *see* Intracranial pressure, raised
Hypoalbuminaemia, 223
Hypocalcaemia, seizures in, 107
Hypogammaglobulinaemia, X-linked, 243
Hypoglycaemia induced by insulin injection, test employing, 251
Hypomagnesaemia, seizures in, 107
Hyponatraemia, seizures in, 107
Hyponatraemic dehydration, 13
Hypopituitarism, neonatal jaundice due to, 225
Hypoproteinaemia, 93–4
Hypothalamo-pituitary-gonadal axis, puberty and, 127–8
Hypothyroidism
  neonatal jaundice due to, 224
  precocious puberty in, 129
Hysterical dyspnoea
  management, 64
  signs/symptoms, 61

Ibuprofen in febrile illness, 69
Imaging, *see* Radiology
Immersion in hot water, deliberate, 39
Immunisation history, 240
Immunodeficiency, 240–4
  acquired (syndrome), 241–4

severe combined, 243
Immunoglobulin A deficiency, 243
Immunoglobulin levels in autoimmune chronic active hepatitis, 84
Infant(s), *see also* Toddlers
constipation, 157–8
death, sudden, *see* Sudden infant death
fever, 66–9
newborn, *see* Neonates
skin conditions/rashes, 257, 258
vomiting, 21–3
Infanticide, 116
Infection(s), 238–44, *see also specific infectious conditions and (types of) pathogens*
bone/joint, limping with, 87, 89
cholestasis due to, 219
chronic/recurrent, 238–44
short stature due to, 248
diarrhoea due to, 9–10
ear, 240
fever with, 69
in headache, examination for sites of, 200
jaundice due to, 78, 224
respiratory/chest
asthma exacerbated by, 238–40
coughing with, 47–8
in cystic fibrosis, 163, 166–7
dyspnoea with, 58–9
stridor with, 121
seizures due to, 108, 110–11
skin, 240, 258, 259, 259–60
urinary tract, 75, 240
Inflammatory bowel diseases, 152–3
Inflammatory skin conditions, 258
Information on poisoning, 100
Informing the patient/parents, 5–6
Inhaled medication in asthma, 138, 139–40
Injury/trauma
bleeding/bruising due to, 25, 26
non-accidental, *see* Non-accidental injury
Inspiration, obstructed, sound of, 119–23
Insulin, children using, 176, 177
Insulin hypoglycaemia test, 251
Interstitial fluid, excessive, *see* Oedema
Interstitial pneumonitis, lymphocytic, 244
Intestine/bowel, *see also specific regions*
inflammatory disease, 152–3
intussusception, 22
obstruction, 22, 23
volvulus, 22
vomiting due to problems in, 22, 23
Intracranial injuries, non-accidental, 38
Intracranial pathology, precocious puberty due to, 129
Intracranial pressure, raised, 109, 110
causes, 202
investigations, 203
management, 109
seizures due to, 109, 110
vomiting due to, 21, 23
Intracranial tumours, 202
Intravenous fluid therapy
in diarrhoeal illness, 14, 15
in shock, 34
Intussusception, 22
Investigations, general aspects, 4–5
Ipecac(uanha) in poisoning, 99, 100
Iron deficiency
anaemia of, 230, 231
infantile, 158
Irritable hip, 87–8
Isotopic imaging, *see* Radionuclide imaging

Jaundice, 77–86, 217–28
causes, 78
neonatal, 217–28
Jitteriness, 194
Joint problems, limping with, 87, 89

Kartagener's syndrome, 50
Kasai operation, 226
Kayser–Fleischer rings, 80
Kidney
calculi, 75
disease (in general)
albuminuria/proteinuria in, 94

failure to thrive due to, 190
haematuria in, 74, 75
tests, in liver disease, 81
Klinefelter's syndrome, delayed puberty in, 132

Lactase deficiency, *see* Lactose, intolerance
Lactose, intolerance (lactase deficiency), 234, 237
transient, 151
Lactose-free food in diarrhoeal illness, 14
Language problems, 174
Laparotomy in biliary disease, diagnostic, 226
Laryngomalacia, 120
Laryngotracheobronchitis, 121, 122
Laxatives, 161–2
Learning difficulties (mental handicap/retardation), 171, 173
constipation in children with, 162
diagnosis, 173
Leptospirosis, 83
Leukaemia, meningeal, 202
Life-threatening events, apparent, 116–18, 195
Limping child, 87–90
'no diagnosis', 90
Lipoprotein, liver-specific, autoantibodies to, 84
Liver, 77–86, 217–28
biopsy, 85, 225–6
disease, 77–86, 217–28
failure to thrive due to, 190
neonatal, 217–28
tests/profile, 81
transplantation, 86
ultrasonography, 84, 225
Liver-specific lipoprotein, autoantibodies to, 84
Lumbar puncture, 67–9, 108
meningitis and, 69, 108, 200–1
Lung function tests in dyspnoea, 62, *see also* Respiratory tract
Lymphocyte abnormalities, 241, 242
Lymphocytic interstitial pneumonitis, 244

McCune–Albright syndrome, precocious puberty in, 129
Macrocytic anaemia, 231
Macule, definition, 255
Magnesium blood levels, seizures with low, 107
Magnetic resonance imaging, seizure patient, 196
Malabsorption
cystic fibrosis, 167
failure to thrive associated with, 189
hypoproteinaemic oedema associated with, 93–4
short stature due to, 248
Malnutrition, *see* Nutrition
Mannitol therapy, 110
Masturbatory movements in toddlers, 195
Meadow's syndrome (Munchausen's syndrome by proxy), poisoning in, 41
Meningeal leukaemia, 202
Meningism, 200
Meningitis
investigations, 69, 200–1
management, 111
seizures in, 108, 111
Meningococcal septicaemia, 26
Mental handicap/retardation, *see* Learning difficulties
Metabolic disease, inherited (inborn errors), *see also specific diseases*
jaundice in, 78, 224
vomiting with, 20
Metered dose inhalers, 139, 140
Microbiology (bacteriology/virology)
diarrhoeal illness, 13, 154
seizure patients, 108
Micturition, involuntary nocturnal, *see* Enuresis
Migraine, 23, 201–2, 203, 235–6
abdominal, 235–6
vomiting with, 23
Milia, 258
Minerals, blood levels, seizure patient, 107, *see also specific minerals*
Mitral valve lesions, 208, 212

Molluscum contagiosum, 259
Mortalities, *see* Infanticide; Sudden infant death
Motor development, delayed, 173–4
Munchausen's syndrome by proxy, poisoning in, 41
Murmurs, 205–16
  exercise-related responses, 213
  frequency, 209
  intensity, 210
    site of maximum, 209
  posture affecting, 211–12
  quality, 211
  radiation, 211
  respiration affecting, 212–13
  timing, 207–9
  Valsalva manoeuvre-related response, 213
Mycoplasma pneumoniae, 63
Myocardiopathy, obstructive, *see* Cardiomyopathy, obstructive
Myocarditis
  management, 64
  symptoms, 61
Myoclonus, 194
  neonatal sleep, 194

Naevi, spider, 79
Naloxone in opiate poisoning, 100
Napkin rash, 258
Nebulisers in asthma, 139
Neglect, 41
Neonates
  cholestasis, 217–28
  constipation, 156–7, 157
  haematuria, 74
  rash (chronic), 258
  sleep myoclonus, 194
  vitamin K prophylaxis, 30
Nervous system, *see also entries under* Neurological *and parts of nervous system*
Neurological disorders
  collapse due to, 35
  constipation due to, 159, 160
  failure to thrive due to, 189
  vomiting due to, 21, 22
Neurological examination
  headache, 203
  seizures, 106
  vomiting child, 20
Newborn, vitamin K prophylaxis, 30
Night-time
  enuresis, *see* Enuresis
  terrors, 145
  waking, 145
Nocturnal disorders, *see* Night-time
Non-accidental injury (physical abuse), 37–45
  bleeding with, 25, 26
  bruising with, 25, 26, 38–9
  conditions mimicking, 39
Normoglycaemia, maintenance, 176
Nutrition/diet, *see also* Eating; Feeding
  compliance with, in diabetes, 177
  management
    in cholestatic neonates, 226–7
    in cystic fibrosis, 167
    in diarrhoeal illness, 14–16
  poor (undernutrition/malnutrition)
    abdominal pain due to, 234
    constipation in neonates due to, 158
    diarrhoeal illness due to, 157–8
    failure to thrive due to, 189
    iron-deficiency anaemia due to, 230, 231
    short stature due to, 248

Obstruction
  airway, stridor due to, 119–23
  biliary, extrahepatic, 219
  intestinal, 22, 23
  ventricular outflow tract, 210
Obstructive cardiomyopathy, *see* Cardiomyopathy, obstructive
Ocular signs/symptoms in jaundice/hepatobiliary disease, 80, 220, 222
Oedema, 91–5
  generalised, 93
  local, 93
Oesophageal reflux, *see* Reflux
Oesophagotracheal fistula, 48, 50
Ophthalmological signs/symptoms in jaundice/hepatobiliary disease, 80, 220, 222

Opiates
in diarrhoeal illness, 16
poisoning, 100
Oral rehydration therapy in diarrhoeal illness, 14, 15
Osteomyelitis, 89
Otitis media, 240
Oxygen therapy in dyspnoea, 63

Pain, abdominal, 233–7
Pallor, 229–32
Pansystolic murmurs, 208, 211
Papilloma virus, 259
Papule, definition, 255
Paracetamol (acetaminophen)
in febrile illness, 69
poisoning, 100–2
Parasitic infection, diarrhoea due to, 10
Parents
of crying child, gaining trust and co-operation, 54
education, *see* Education
height, 247
informing, 6
reaction to stimulation by, on Acute Illness Observation Scale, 68
of seizure patient, 110
stress in, infantile colic and, association between, 56
in sudden infant death, 114–15
Peptic ulcer, 234
Pericardial effusions, 61
Periodic syndrome, 235–6
Pertussis, 47–8
Petechiae/petechial rash, 26–7
definition, 255
Petit mal, 193
Phagocyte deficiencies, 242, 243
Phenobarbitone with seizures, 109
Phenothiazine poisoning, 100
Phenytoin with seizures, 109
Physical abuse, *see* Non-accidental injury
Physostigmine salicylate, 102
Pituitary dysfunction, neonatal jaundice due to, 225, *see also* Hypothalamo-pituitary-gonadal axis
Pityrosporum ovale, 258
Place of Safety Order, 44
Plain films, *see* X-rays
Plantar dermatosis, 260
Pneumococcal pneumonia, 63
Pneumonia
management, 63
signs/symptoms, 47, 60, 70
Pneumonitis, lymphocytic interstitial, 244
Poisoning, 96–102
drug, 96–102
non-accidental/intentional, 41, 97
vomiting caused by, 23, 98
food, toxin-mediated, 10
Portoenterostomy, hepatic, 226
Precocious puberty, 128–32
Pregnancy, failure to thrive and effects of, 187
Premature puberty, 128–32
Presystolic murmur, 208
Protection of abused child, 43–4
Protein(s)
low blood/serum levels, *see* Hypoalbuminaemia; Hypoproteinaemia
synthesis, failure, 94
Protein-losing enteropathies, 94
Proteinuria, 94
Protozoan infections, diarrhoeal illness with, 10, 151
management, 16
Pruritus in cholestatic neonates, 227
Pseudomonas aeruginosa and *P. cepacia* infection in cystic fibrosis, 163, 166
Psoriasis, 260
Psychogenic abdominal pain, 236, 237
Psychogenic coughing, 49
Psychosocial problems, short stature due to, 248, 252
Puberty, 127–36
delayed, 132
endocrinology, 127–8
precocious, 128–32
Pulmonary function tests in dyspnoea, 62, *see also* Respiratory tract

Pulmonary valve lesions, 207, 208, 210
Punishment with behavioural problems, 142
Purpura, 26–7, 27–8, 257
Pyloric stenosis, 22–3
Pyrexia, *see* Fever

Quadriplegia, 174

Radiology, *see also specific methods*
  delayed puberty, 133
  in hepatobiliary disease, 81, 84–5, 222, 225
  limping child, 89
  precocious puberty, 130
  seizure patient, 109
Radionuclide/isotopic imaging (scintigraphy)
  bone, limping child, 89
  hepatobiliary, neonatal, 225
Rash, skin, 255–61
  acute, 255–7
  chronic, 257–60
  seizure patients with, 106–7
Rectal examination in constipation, 160
Reflex anal dilatation, 160
Reflex anoxic events, 194
Reflux, gastro-oesophageal, 22
  cough in, 48, 50
  investigations, 50
Rehydration therapy in diarrhoeal illness, 14, 15
Renal disease, *see* Kidney
Respiration, murmurs in response to, 212–13
Respiratory distress, chronic, 190
Respiratory failure, acute, collapse due to, 35
Respiratory monitors in sudden infant death-risk children, 115
Respiratory tract disorders/disease, *see also* Lung
  cough due to, 47–8
  in cystic fibrosis, 163–4
  dyspnoea in, 58–60
  infectious, *see* Infection
  stridor due to, 120, 121, 122
Resuscitation, *see also* First aid
  collapsed child, 32–3
  poisoning, 98–9
  seizures, 105
Reye's syndrome, 21
Ringworm (tinea), 259–60
Rotavirus-related diarrhoea, 9

Scabies, 259
Scalds, non-accidental, 39
Scintigraphy, *see* Radionuclide imaging
Seborrhoeic dermatitis, 258
Seizures/fits/convulsions, 103–11, 192–8
  acute presentation, 103–11
  causes, 103
  outpatient management, 192–8
Sepsis, bacterial, 67
Septic arthritis, 89
Septicaemia, meningococcal, 26
Septo-optic dysplasia, 225
Sex hormones, precocious puberty caused by ingestion, 129
Sex-linked hypogammaglobulinaemia, 243
Sexual abuse, 42–3, 44, 160
Sexual development at puberty, 127–36
  abnormal, 127–36
  normal, 127–8
Shake injuries, 38
Shock, management, 33–5
Short-gut syndrome, 187
Short stature, *see* Stature
SIDS, *see* Sudden infant death syndrome
Skeletal dysplasia, 248
Skin
  infections, 240, 258, 259, 259–60
  in jaundice/hepatobiliary disease, signs, 80, 221
  pale colour, 229–32
  prick tests, in asthma, 137–8
  rash, *see* Rash
Skinfold thickness, measurement, 246
Skull fractures, non-accidental, 38, *see also entries under* Intracranial
Sleep myoclonus, neonatal, 194

Sleeping problems, 144–5
Smacking, 142
Social approach, response to, on Acute Illness Observation Scale, status, 68
Social behaviour, abnormal, 146–7
Social factors
  failure to thrive related to, 187–8, 190
  short stature related to, 248, 252
Sodium (ion), abnormal levels, *see* Hypernatraemia; Hyponatraemia
Sodium cromoglycate in asthma, 138, 139
Sodium valproate with seizures, 109
Sonography, *see* Ultrasonography
Sounds, heart, 206–7
Spastic diplegia, 174
Spider naevi, 79
Spinal cord problems, constipation due to, 159
Spleen
  absence, 243
  ultrasonography in hepatobiliary disease, 84, 225
Stature, short, 245–54
  causes, 248–9, 249
    normal, 248, 249
    pathological, 248–9, 249
  definition, 245–6
Stenosis
  aortic (valve), 208, 209, 211
  mitral, 208
  pulmonary, 207, 208
  pyloric, 22–3
Steroids
  in asthma
    inhaled, 138, 139
    oral, 138
  in cystic fibrosis, 167
Stethoscope in cardiac auscultation, 206, 209
Stomach emptying in poisoning, 98, 99–100, *see also entries under* Gastroenteritis
Stones (calculi), renal, 75
Stools/faeces, analysis
  in diarrhoeal illness, 13, 154
  in jaundice/liver disease, 80
Stress, parental, colic and, association between, 56
Stridor, 119–23
Sudden infant death syndrome (SIDS), 112–16
  aetiology/risk factors, 115, 115–16
  management, 113–14
  monitoring children at risk of, 115
  near-miss (apparent life-threatening events), 116–18
  recurrence, 114–15
Sugar/glucose, blood, seizure patient, 107
Supraventricular tachycardia, *see* Tachycardia
Sweat test, 224
Syncope, 195
Synovitis, irritable, 87–8
Systolic murmurs, 207–8
  diastolic and, 208
  ejection, 210, 211

T cell deficiency, 241, 242, 243
Tachycardia, supraventricular
  management, 64
  symptoms, 61
Tantrums, temper, 146
Technetium bone scans, limping child, 89
Teenagers, *see* Adolescents
Temper tantrums, 146
Temperature, body, abnormally high, *see* Fever
Teratoma, presacral, 160
Tests, value of, 4–5, *see also specific tests*
Tetany, 195
Tetralogy of Fallot, 208
Thelarche, premature, 131
Theophyllines in asthma, 139
Thiopentone with seizures, 109
Thrive, failure to, 40–1, 186–91
Thrombocytopenia, causes, 29, 29–30
Thyroid dysfunction
  neonatal jaundice due to, 224
  precocious puberty due to, 129
Tics, 195
Tinea, 259–60
Toddlers, *see also* Infants

constipation, 158
diarrhoea, 151
fever, 66–9
limping, 87–9
Toxicology, *see* Poisoning
Toxin-mediated food poisoning, 10
Tracheitis, bacterial, 121
Tracheo-oesophageal fistula, 48, 50
Tranquilliser poisoning, 98
Transaminase (aminotransferase) levels, 81–2, 221–3
Transplantation, liver, 86
Trauma, *see* Injury
Tricuspid valve lesions, 212–13
Trust, gaining
of crying child, 54
of parents of crying child, 54
Tuberculosis, coughing, 48
Tumours
gonadotrophin-producing, precocious puberty caused by, 129
intracranial, 202
Turner's syndrome (XO), delayed puberty in, 132
Tyrosinaemia, 224

Ulcer, peptic, 234
Ulcerative colitis, 152
Ultrasonography
cardiac, 214
in hepatobiliary disease, 84, 225
Undernutrition, *see* Nutrition
Urea, blood, seizure patient, 107
Urinary tract infection, 75, 240
Urine
albumin in, excess, 94
blood in, *see* Haematuria
examination/analysis, 73
in jaundice/liver disease, 80, 222
output in diarrhoeal illness, 13
protein in, excess, 94
Urticaria, 257, 258

Valproate with seizures, 109
Valsalva manoeuvre, murmurs in response to, 213
Vascular access in collapsed child, 33, *see also* Arteries; Veins
Veins
access in collapsed child, 33
fluid therapy via, *see* Intravenous fluid therapy
Ventricles
outflow ejection murmur, left, 212
outflow tract obstructive lesions, 210
septal defect, 208, 209, 211
Vesicle, definition, 255
Viral infection
diarrhoea due to, 9, 10
diagnosis, 13
hepatitis caused by, *see* Hepatitis
pneumonia caused by, 47
Virology, *see* Microbiology
Vitamin K prophylaxis of newborn, 30
Volvulus, midgut, 22–3
Vomiting, 18–24
cause(s) of, 18, 19, 98
poisoning as, 23, 98
cough (chronic) and, 48
induced, in cases of poisoning, 98, 99–100
Vulvovaginitis, 234–5

Waking at night, 145
Warts, 259
Weight in growth assessment, 246
Whooping cough (pertussis), 47–8
Wilson's disease, 83, 85–6

X-linked hypogammaglobulinaemia, 243
XO (Turner's) syndrome, delayed puberty in, 132
X-rays, plain film
constipation, 160–1
heart murmurs, 214
limping child, 89
seizure patient, 109
XXY (Klinefelter's) syndrome, delayed puberty in, 132